Techniques in Interventional Radiology

Other titles in this Series

Timothy Clark • Tarun Sabharwal
Editors

Michael J. Lee • Anthony F. Watkinson
Series Editors

Interventional Radiology Techniques in Ablation

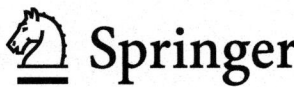 Springer

Editors
Timothy Clark, MD, FSIR
Department of Radiology
Section of Vascular
and Interventional Radiology
University of Pennsylvania
Philadelphia, PA
USA

Tarun Sabharwal, MB,ChB, FRCSI, FRCR
Department of Radiology
St Thomas' Hospital
London
UK

Series Editors
Michael J. Lee, MSc, FRCPI, FRCR,
FFR(RCSI), FSIR, EBIR
Department of Radiology
Beaumont Hospital
Dublin
Ireland

Anthony F. Watkinson, BSc, MSc(oxon),
MBBS, FRCS, FRCR, EBIR
Department of Radiology
The Royal Devon and Exeter Hospital
and Peninsula Medical School
Exeter
UK

ISBN 978-0-85729-093-9   ISBN 978-0-85729-094-6   (eBook)
DOI 10.1007/978-0-85729-094-6
Springer Dordrecht Heidelberg New York London

Library of Congress Control Number: 2012948088

Preface from the Series Editors

Interventional radiology treatments now play a major role in many disease processes and continue to mushroom with novel procedures appearing almost on a yearly basis. Indeed, it is becoming more and more difficult to be an expert in all facets of interventional radiology. The interventional trainee and practising interventional radiologist will have to attend meetings and read extensively to keep up to date. There are many IR textbooks that are disease specific, but incorporate interventional radiology techniques. These books are important to understand the natural history, epidemiology, pathophysiology, and diagnosis of disease processes. However, a detailed handbook that is technique-based is a useful addition to have in the Cath Lab, office, or at home where information can be accessed quickly, before, or even during a case. With this in mind we have embarked on a series of books which will provide technique-specific information on IR procedures. Initialy, technique handbooks on angioplasty and stenting, transcatheter embolization, biopsy and drainage and ablative techniques will comprise the series. In the future we hope to add books on pediatric and neurointervention.

We have chosen two editors, who are expert in their fields, for each book. One editor is an European and the other is an American so that the knowledge of detailed IR techniques is balanced and representative. We have tried to make the information easy to access using a consistent bullet point format with sections on clinical features, anatomy, tools, patient preparation, technique, aftercare, complications, and key points at the end of each chapter.

These technique-specific books will be of benefit to those residents and fellows who are training in interventional radiology and who may be taking subspeciality certificate examinations in interventional radiology. In addition, these books will be of help to most practicing interventional radiologists in academic or private practice. We hope that these books will be left in the interventional lab where they should also be of benefit to ancillary staff, such as radiology technicians, radiographers, or nurses who are specializing in the care of patients referred to interventional radiology.

We hope that you will use these books extensively and that they will be of help during your working IR career.

Dublin, Ireland   Michael J. Lee
Exeter, UK   Anthony F. Watkinson

Preface

In preparing *Interventional Radiology Techniques in Ablation* we sought to develop a practical and concise guide to contemporary techniques in image-guided tumor ablation. This handbook is intended to serve as a quick reference for physicians in interventional radiology training as well as a resource for IR technologists, nurses, nurse practitioners, and physician assistants.

To avoid duplicate descriptions of ablation technologies within multiple clinical applications, we have divided the book into a Technology Overview section addressing current ablation technologies followed by chapters addressing specific clinical applications. We have utilized the expertise of contributors from the USA, Europe, and Asia to provide broad and international perspectives on tumor ablation. This includes chapters on well-established applications such as liver ablation to more recent developments in breast and endocrine ablation. We have retained the style of this series, with consistent headings across chapters to provide organization for general reading and enable rapid access to key points. Each chapter is supplemented with a short list of up-to-date references to serve as the basis for further reading. Selected figures are provided to illustrate important concepts.

We are grateful to Professors Lee and Watkinson for their vision and guidance in the development of this unique series. We are also very appreciative of the patience and support of Springer-Verlag, particularly Maureen Alexander.

Timothy Clark
Tarun Sabharwal

Contents

Contributors

Irfan Ahmed, M.B.B.S., MRCP, FRCR Department of Radiology, Guy's and St Thomas' Foundation Trust, St Thomas' Hospital, London, UK

Jung Hwan Baek, M.D. Department of Radiology and Research Institute of Radiology, University of Ulsan College of Medicine, Asan Medical Center, Seoul, South Korea

Michael D. Beland, M.D. Department of Diagnostic Imaging, Rhode Island Hospital, The Warren Alpert Medical School of Brown University, Providence, RI, USA

Rachel R Bitton, Ph.D. Department of Radiology, Lucas Center for Imaging, Stanford University, School of Medicine, Stanford, CA, USA

Chris L. Brace, Ph.D. Department of Radiology, University of Wisconsin, School of Medicine and Public Health, Madison, WI, USA

Department of Radiology, University of Wisconsin Hospital and Clinics, Madison, WI, USA

Departments of Biomedical Engineering and Medical Physics, University of Wisconsin, School of Medicine and Public Health, Madison, WI, USA

Daniel B. Brown, M.D. Division of Interventional Radiology, Department of Radiology, Thomas Jefferson University, Philadelphia, PA, USA

Timothy Clark, M.D., FSIR Department of Radiology, Section of Vascular and Interventional Radiology, University of Pennsylvania, Philadelphia, PA, USA

Xavier Buy, M.D. Department of Interventional Radiology, University Hospital of Strasbourg, Strasbourg, France

Bruce L. Daniel, M.D. Department of Radiology, Stanford University, School of Medicine, Stanford, CA, USA

Iulian Enescu, M.D. Department of Interventional Radiology, University Hospital of Strasbourg, Strasbourg, France

Joseph P. Erinjeri, M.D., Ph.D. Interventional Radiology Service, Memorial Sloan-Kettering Cancer Center, New York, NY, USA

Department of Radiology, Weill Cornell Medical College, New York, USA

Nicos Fotiadis, M.D., FRCR Department of Interventional Oncology, The Royal Marsden NHS Foundation Trust, London, UK

Department of Interventional Radiology, St Bartholomew's & The Royal London Hospitals, London, UK

Afshin Gangi, M.D., Ph.D. Department of Interventional Radiology, University Hospital of Strasbourg, Strasbourg, France

Department of Non-vascular Interventional Radiology, University Hospital of Strasbourg, Strasbourg, France

Julien Garnon, M.D. Department of Interventional Radiology, University Hospital of Strasbourg, Strasbourg, France

J. Louis Hinshaw, M.D. Department of Radiology, University of Wisconsin, School of Medicine and Public Health, Madison, WI, USA

Department of Radiology, University of Wisconsin Hospital and Clinics, Madison, WI, USA

Jeffrey A. Klein, M.D. Department of Radiology, University of Wisconsin, School of Medicine and Public Health, Madison, WI, USA

Department of Radiology, University of Wisconsin Hospital and Clinics, Madison, WI, USA

Katsanos Konstantinos, M.D., Ph.D., EBIR Department of Interventional Radiology, Patras University Hospital (PGNP), Rion, Patras, Greece

Miltiadis Krokidis, M.D., Ph.D., EBIR Department of Radiology, Guy's and St Thomas' Foundation Trust, St Thomas' Hospital, London, UK

Hervé Lang, M.D., Ph.D. Urology Department, University Hospital of Strasbourg, Strasbourg, France

Fred T. Lee, M.D. Department of Radiology, University of Wisconsin, School of Medicine and Public Health, Madison, WI, USA

Department of Radiology, University of Wisconsin Hospital and Clinics, Madison, WI, USA

Meghan G. Lubner, M.D. Department of Radiology, University of Wisconsin, School of Medicine and Public Health, Madison, WI, USA

Department of Radiology, University of Wisconsin Hospital and Clinics, Madison, WI, USA

William W. Mayo-Smith, M.D. Department of Diagnostic Imaging, Rhode Island Hospital, The Warren Alpert Medical School of Brown University, Providence, RI, USA

Kim R. Butts Pauly, Ph.D. Department of Radiology, Lucas Center for Imaging, Stanford University, School of Medicine, Stanford, CA, USA

Theodore Petsas, M.D., Ph.D. Department of Interventional Radiology, Patras University Hospital (PGNP), Rion, Patras, Greece

Shuvro Roy-Choudhury Diagnostic and Interventional Radiology, Fortis Hospitals, Kolkata, West Bengal, India

Consultant Radiologist, Heart of England NHS Foundation Trust, Birmingham, UK

Georgia Tsoumakidou, M.D. Department of Interventional Radiology, University Hospital of Strasbourg, Strasbourg, France

Department of Non-vascular Interventional Radiology, University Hospital of Strasbourg, Strasbourg, France

Department of Urology, University Hospital of Strasbourg, Strasbourg, France

Ronald S. Winokur, M.D. Division of Interventional Radiology, Department of Radiology, Thomas Jefferson University Hospital, Philadelphia, PA, USA

Chapter 1
Introduction

Timothy Clark

The last 30 years have witnessed the emergence of a new clinical subspecialty in the war against cancer – that of interventional oncology. Armed with ablation devices, embolization agents, cytotoxic and radiotherapeutic agents, intravascular delivery systems, and advances in imaging guidance, interventional oncologists have evolved into a fourth pivotal member complementing the cancer-treating trifecta of medical, surgical, and radiation oncologists. Interventional oncology is rapidly changing the paradigm of modern cancer management by improving local control and even cure of many solid organ malignancies. Image-guided tumor ablation is a fundamental tool within the therapeutic array of the interventional oncologist and is the focus of this book.

We have designed this book to be as practical as possible. It is organized to cover the major ablation technologies in current clinical use in Technology Overview, followed by Clinical Applications with an organ-based description of clinical applications of image-guided ablation in the field of interventional oncology.

Leading off for the Technology Overview section of this book, Drs. Krokidis and Ahmed in Chap. 2 provide insight into the mechanism of radiofrequency ablation, information on electrode selection, and practical suggestions when using each of the most widely used commercially available systems. Chapter 3 by Dr. Erinjeri addresses cryoablation, including its mechanism of tumor destruction, components required, and advantages and disadvantages. In Chap. 4, Dr. Klein et al. discuss microwave systems for tumor ablation, including mechanisms, components, advantages/disadvantages, and future directions. Chapter 5 by Dr. Garnon et al. covers high-intensity focused ultrasound, laser interstitial ablation, and chemical ablation.

T. Clark, M.D., FSIR
Department of Radiology, Section of Vascular and Interventional Radiology,
Penn Presbyterian Medical Center and University of Pennsylvania Medical Center,
39th and Market Streets, Philadelphia, PA 19104, USA
e-mail: timothy.clark@uphs.upenn.edu

T. Clark, T. Sabharwal (eds.), *Interventional Radiology Techniques in Ablation*,
Techniques in Interventional Radiology,
DOI 10.1007/978-0-85729-094-6_1, © Springer-Verlag London 2013

Chapter 6 by Dr. Konstantinos completes the Technology Overview section of the book with a discussion of plasma-mediated coblation.

The Clinical Application section of the book takes a head-to-toe approach, and begins in Chap. 7 with a description of ablation of thyroid and parathyroid nodules by Dr. Baek. Chapter 8 by Drs. Bitton, Daniel, and Pauly addresses thermal ablation of breast carcinoma and fibroadenomas, a field that is expected to significantly grow given the high incidence and prevalence of breast cancer. In Chap. 9, Dr. Roy-Chourhury describes the role and technique of lung tumor ablation, also expected to experience significant growth given the epidemiology of primary lung carcinoma and lung metastases. Drs. Winokur and Brown discuss thermal ablation of hepatocellular carcinoma and liver metastases in Chap. 10, which remains the clinical application of thermal ablation with the broadest worldwide experience. Chapter 11 by Dr. Fotiadis addresses thermal ablation of renal carcinoma, with unique considerations in that most patients are treated with a completely curative intent. Chapter 12 by Drs. Beland and Mayo-Smith describe the use of thermal ablation of primary adrenal tumors and adrenal neoplasms, including the need for preprocedural alpha and beta blockade for functioning adrenal tumors. In Chap. 13, Drs. Tsoumakidou, Lang, and Gangi discuss the evolving role of thermal ablation for treatment of prostate carcinoma, which is expected to extend the spectrum of patients in whom local tumor control can be achieved. Finally, Chap. 14 by Drs. Konstantinos and Petsas completes this book with a description of ablation of primary bone and soft tissue tumors.

Tumor ablation is a rapidly evolving field, both with emerging technologies and new clinical applications. Some newer ablation technologies, such as irreversible electroporation, have had insufficient clinical experience at the time of publication and are not addressed in the book; a number of these ablation modalities hold exciting promise and their omission in this book should not be interpreted as an assessment of their clinical potential. Similarly, the use of image-guided ablation in diseases such as pancreatic adenocarcinoma is not addressed, as only preliminary clinical data exist for these applications at present. We have also not addressed the evolving technologies in image fusion, navigation, and robotic systems, which are expected to enable tumor ablation to become safer, more precise, and faster.

We hope that you find this handbook practical, well-organized, and clinically relevant.

Part I
Technology Assessment

Chapter 2
Overview of Thermal Ablation Devices: Radiofrequency Ablation

Miltiadis Krokidis and Irfan Ahmed

Background

- "Thermal ablation" is defined as the application of heating agents to a specific area of the body with the intention of tissue destruction.
- The deleterious effect of heat is based on the fact that when biological tissues reach a temperature above 45°C, irreversible cell damage occurs.
- Radiofrequency (RF) ablation is based on the interaction between high-frequency, rapidly alternating electric current and biological tissue.
- The rapidly alternating electric current causes vibration movement of the tissue's bipolar molecules (mostly water).
- This vibration movement is transmitted between adjacent molecules with resulting frictional energy loss.
- The energy loss is deposited in the biological tissues in the form of a rise in temperature.
- The rise in temperature leads initially to hyperthermia and then to "coagulation" necrosis.

Basic Principles

- In RF ablation, necrosis is achieved with electromagnetic energy sources in the range of 375–500 kHz.
- Available devices may be either monopolar or bipolar systems.

M. Krokidis, M.D., Ph.D., EBIR (✉) • I. Ahmed, M.B.B.S., MRCP, FRCR
Department of Radiology, Guy's and St Thomas' NHS Trust, St Thomas' Hospital,
1st Floor Lambeth Wing, Westminster Bridge Road, London SE1 7EH, UK
e-mail: miltiadis.krokidis@gstt.nhs.uk, mkrokidis@hotmail.com; irfan.ahmed@gstt.nhs.uk

T. Clark, T. Sabharwal (eds.), *Interventional Radiology Techniques in Ablation*,
Techniques in Interventional Radiology,
DOI 10.1007/978-0-85729-094-6_2, © Springer-Verlag London 2013

- There are a variety of available electrodes (multitined, expandable, internally cooled, and perfusion electrodes).
- In the RF ablation circuit, the (monopolar) electrode acts as the cathode and the pads as the anode.
- The electrode tip concentrates high energy in a small area and the grounding pads disperse that energy due to the larger area.
- There is a different algorithm used for each RF ablation application (ramped energy deposition or impedance regulated).
- There are different ablation protocol types (time, use of isolating or ablation-enhancing agents) that vary according to the target organ.
- The main limitation of RF ablation is that it depends on the appropriate thermal conductivity of the surrounding tissues.
- Desiccated tissue around the electrode acts as an insulating agent and limits thermal energy transmission.
- If the temperature rapidly reaches above 100°C, then boiling, vaporization, and carbonization occur, all of which decrease energy transmission and limit the ablation effect.
- The objective is to heat the surrounding tissues between 50°C and 100°C for more than 9 min without causing charring or vaporization.
- To avoid tissue desiccation (charring) and vaporization, gradual tissue energy deposition needs to be performed.
- A 1-cm "ablation margin" is necessary around the treated lesion to cover microscopic tumor extension.
- The effectiveness of the ablation process is also limited by the "heat sink" effect due to the presence of adjacent blood vessels.
- The development of a thermal lesion is described by the following relationship: induced coagulation necrosis = (energy deposited × local tissue interactions) – heat loss.
- The temperature of the surrounding tissues is inversely proportional to the distance from the tip of the electrode. The relationship is described by the following equation: $T = 1/r^4$ where T is the temperature and r is the radius around the electrode.
- There is a limited area of 2.2–2.4 cm of ablation around a single needle-like electrode.
- The ablation process may be enhanced by (a) improving the conduction of thermal energy, (b) decreasing the heat tolerance of the tumor, and (c) increasing the energy deposition.

Types of Electrodes

- The RF electrode has an insulated shaft and a noninsulated active tip, which is in contact with the lesion.
- Initially electrodes were single and straight offering a cylindrical ablation zone.
- Electrode shape modification to a central cannula and multiple externally curved noninsulated extensions in the shape of an umbrella then occurred.

- This umbrella shape resulted in a larger and more reproducible ablation zone.
- To reduce tissue charring, internally cooled electrodes were also developed.
- Further electrode modifications include the ability to inject or to infuse saline solution in the ablation zone aiming to expand the ablation zone.
- There is no significant difference demonstrated thus far in the results offered by the different electrodes and it has been shown that the result of RF ablation mainly depends on the operator's experience and the size of the tumor.
- Bipolar ablation systems have also recently been developed.
- In bipolar systems, the applied RF current is addressed from one electrode directly to another without closing the circuit with the use of grounding pads.
- With bipolar systems, large energy dispersion is avoided, but the same physical properties apply to both bipolar and monopolar systems.

Types of Generators

- There are different available RF generators that follow different ablation protocols.
- The main protocols of monopolar systems include impedance control, time, and temperature feedback.
- Bipolar systems use a fixed-energy algorithm that is controlled by the increase in tissue resistance due to desiccation of the target lesion.

Commercially Available RF Systems: Boston Scientific

- The radiofrequency generator manufactured by Boston Scientific (RF 3000, Boston Scientific, Natick, MA) produces alternating current at a frequency of 480 kHz with a maximum power output of 200 W (Fig. 2.1).
- The algorithm used is based on feedback from target tissue impedance.
- Tissue impedance is continuously monitored and the energy output of each electrode is adjusted on the basis of the impedance value.

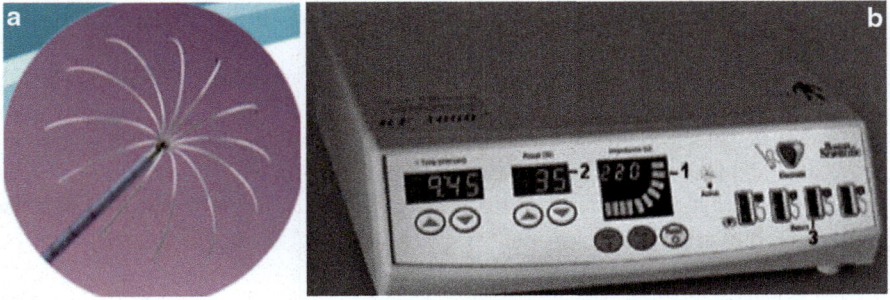

Fig. 2.1 (**a**) LeVeen electrode with umbrella-like deployment configuration (LeVeen; Boston Scientific). (**b**) Boston Scientific RS 3000 RF ablation generator. *1* the value of tissue impedance, *2* the value of the power output in Watts, *3* the Pad-Guard monitor

- The ablation end point is a significant increase in impedance of the ablated tissue.
- The power is increased gradually beginning from 20 to 80 W and then by 5–10 W/min to reach maximum target values of 55–200 W depending on the ablated tissue.
- The manufacturer suggests a second ablation session beginning at 70% of the maximum power.
- The electrode used was introduced by LeVeen and is a monopolar array-type electrode with an umbrella-like deployment configuration (LeVeen; Boston Scientific). The umbrella reaches a diameter of 5 cm.
- The electrodes are 15 gauge and 17 gauge. All electrode tips are active and give impedance feedback.
- Once the electrode is positioned in the target area, the umbrella-like tines are deployed.
- A single straight electrode is also available for small lesions (Soloist electrode).
- A coaxial system is also available from the manufacturer.
- Tract ablation is possible by retracting the prongs and the electrode is subsequently pulled back slowly by continuously applying 30 W.

Commercially Available RF Systems: Covidien

- The Covidien Cool-tip (Boulder, CO; formerly Tyco Healthcare Valleylab) RF Generator (Fig 2.2) produces alternating current with a frequency of 480 kHz offering a power output up to 200 W.
- The generator follows a tissue impedance feedback algorithm with continuous monitoring of tissue impedance, and adjustments are made in order to achieve the appropriate energy output for each electrode.
- The pulsed ablation system allows the tissue to rehydrate during the ablation cycle; tissue impedance is increased gradually and the ablation is more prolonged.
- The electrodes used are straight and monopolar and are cooled internally by saline to enhance slow heating of adjacent tissue.
- Internal cooling reduces charring and vaporization, and thus increases ablation volume and shortens ablation time.
- A cluster electrode is also available that comprises three electrodes all contained within one handle.
- The cluster electrode has up to a 4-cm exposure. Covidien offers four electrode lengths and four tip exposures for customized ablation sizes.
- The needle gauge for the Cool-tip is 17 gauge, and the tip of the electrode is placed optimally slightly beyond the distal margin of the target lesion.

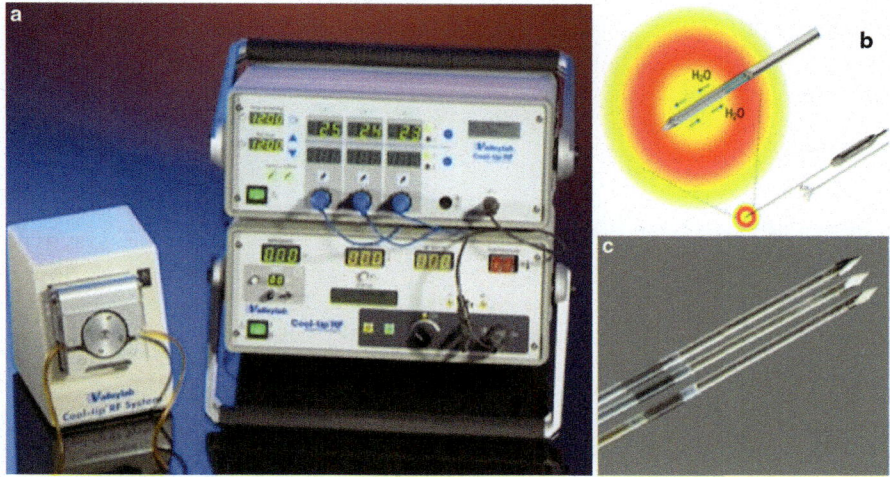

Fig. 2.2 (**a**) Covidien Cool-Tip RF Ablation System; number *1* indicates the infusion pump for the infusion of saline, number *2* is the RF generator and number *3* is the RF switching controller (**b**) A peristaltic pump circulates low temperature saline through the electrode's internal lumen in order to cool the tissue adjacent to the active tip, maintaining a low value of tissue impedance during the ablation cycle thus avoiding a charring effect (**c**) the cluster Cool-Tip electrode

- A Switching Controller is also available with Cool-tip Technology, which allows the use of three separate single electrodes placed simultaneously.
- A tract ablate button is also available when tract ablation is considered necessary.

Commercially Available RF Systems: Angiodynamics

- AngioDynamics RITA medical system uses a 460-kHz generator (Model 1500X, RITA Medical Systems, Mountain View, CA) capable of producing maximum energy output of 250 W (Fig. 2.3).
- The mechanism of ablation is temperature-controlled.
- The tips of the electrodes have thermocouples that report real-time temperature.
- Real-time temperature readings are displayed on the generator console, measured at the five electrode tips.
- RITA has several electrode options with the principal electrode being the Starburst XL electrode, which produces an ablation zone of 3–5 cm. The needle is 15-gauge, and contains nine deployable curved tines.
- When fully extended, the maximum diameter is 5 cm and it mimics the configuration of a Christmas tree.

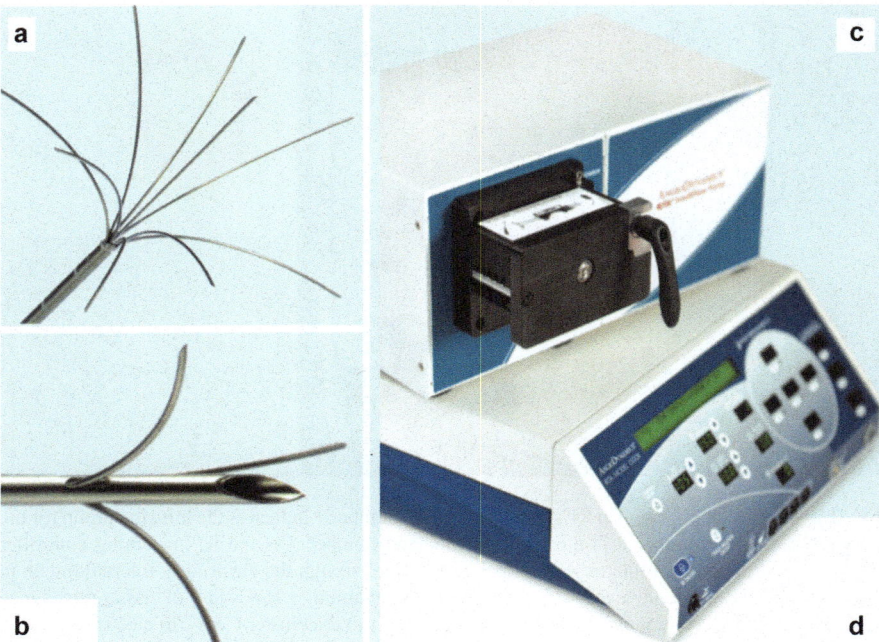

Fig. 2.3 AngioDynamics' StarBurst® radiofrequency ablation system. (**a**) Starburst XL, (**b**) Starburst MRI electrode, (**c**) IntelliFlow pump, and (**d**) Model 1500X RF generator (Photos courtesy of AngioDynamics, Inc.)

- The electrodes are adapted for use in the Computed Tomography gantry (flexible version; SB Flex, SB Semi-Flex) and a Magnetic Resonance Imaging compatible device (SM MRI) is available. There is also a smaller 2-cm device (SB SDE).
- The electrodes need to be deployed at the proximal portion of the target lesion, allowing the tines' tips to form a Christmas tree shape.
- An additional saline infusion system is also available (Intelliflow Pump, Angiodynamics), which infuses saline into the ablation zone.
- Saline infusion enhances ablation effect by reducing charring.
- There are two different saline infusion electrodes (SB XLi-enhanced, for up to 7 cm) and SB Talon with side deployment tines, for difficult access lesions.
- The electrodes may be also placed coaxially.
- When necessary, tract ablation is possible after retracting the prongs and pulling the electrode back slowly with a temperature of 70°C.

Suggested Reading

Ahmed M, Lukyanov AN, Torchilin V, et al. Combined radiofrequency ablation and adjuvant liposomal chemo- therapy: effect of chemotherapeutic agent, nanoparticle size, and circulation time. J Vasc Interv Radiol. 2005a;16(10):1365–71.

Ahmed M, Liu Z, Lukyanov AN, et al. Combination radiofrequency ablation with intratumoral liposomal doxorubicin: effect on drug accumulation and coagulation in multiple tissues and tumor types in animals. Radiology. 2005b;235(2):469–77.

Brown DB, Gould JE, Gervais DA, et al. Transcatheter therapy for hepatic malignancy: standardization of terminology and reporting criteria. J Vasc Interv Radiol. 2007;18(12):1469–78. Review.

Goldberg SN, Gazelle GS, Mueller PR. Thermal ablation therapy for focal malignancy: a unified approach to underlying principles, techniques, and diagnostic imaging guidance. AJR Am J Roentgenol. 2000;174(2):323–31.

LeVeen RF. Laser hyperthermia and radiofrequency ablation of hepatic lesions. Semin Interv Radiol. 1997;14:313–24.

Meijerink MR, van der Tol P, van Tilborg AA. Radiofrequency ablation of large size liver tumors using novel plan-parallel expandable bipolar electrodes: initial clinical experience. Eur J Radiol. 2011;77(1):167–71. Epub ahead of print July 17, 2009.

Organ LW. Electrophysiologic principles of radiofrequency lesion making. Appl Neurophysiol. 1976–1977;39:69–76.

Pereira PL, Trubenbach J, Schenk M, et al. Radiofrequency ablation: in vivo comparison of four commercially available devices in pig livers. Radiology. 2004;232(2):482–90.

Poon RT, Ng KK, Lam CM, et al. Learning curve for radiofrequency ablation of liver tumours: prospective analysis of initial 100 patients in a tertiary institution. Ann Surg. 2004;239(4): 441–9.

Chapter 3
Overview of Thermal Ablation Devices: Cryoablation

Joseph P. Erinjeri

Mechanism of Action

- Cryoablation refers to all methods of destroying tissue by freezing [1]. Cryoablation can be performed via surgical (open or laparoscopic) or percutaneous approaches.
- Percutaneous cryoablation begins with the insertion of a specialized needle (cryoprobe) into malignant tissue under imaging guidance; the needle is then rapidly cooled to subzero temperatures, causing removal of heat from the tissue via conduction.
- Rapid extracellular cooling results in the formation of extracellular ice crystals, which sequesters free water, increasing the tonicity of the extracellular space. Osmotic tension draws free intracellular water from cells, resulting in dehydration [2]. The concomitant increase in intracellular solute concentration results in damage to cytoplasmic enzymes and the destabilization of the cell membrane.
- Rapid intracellular cooling results in intracellular ice crystal formation, a harbinger of lethal cellular injury and subsequent cell [3]. Although the exact mechanism of cellular damage from intracellular ice formation is unknown, injury is thought to be mediated by physical damage to intracellular membranes of organelles and the plasma membrane.
- During thawing, melting ice within the extracellular space results in its hypotonicity with respect to the intracellular compartment. This osmotic gradient can trigger a fluid shift, leading to cell swelling and/or bursting. In addition, an influx

J.P. Erinjeri, M.D., Ph.D.
Interventional Radiology Service, Memorial Sloan Kettering Cancer Center,
1275 York Avenue, New York, NY 10064 , USA

Department of Radiology, Weill Cornell Medical College,
1275 York Avenue, New York, NY 10064, USA
e-mail: erinjerj@mskcc.org

T. Clark, T. Sabharwal (eds.), *Interventional Radiology Techniques in Ablation*,
Techniques in Interventional Radiology,
DOI 10.1007/978-0-85729-094-6_3, © Springer-Verlag London 2013

of free water into the intracellular space provides substrate for the growth of intracellular ice crystals, exacerbating their biocidal effects [4].

• Cellular injury is maximized by optimizing four factors: increasing cooling rate, lowering target temperature, increasing time at target temperature, and decreasing thawing rate [5] (Fig. 3.1).

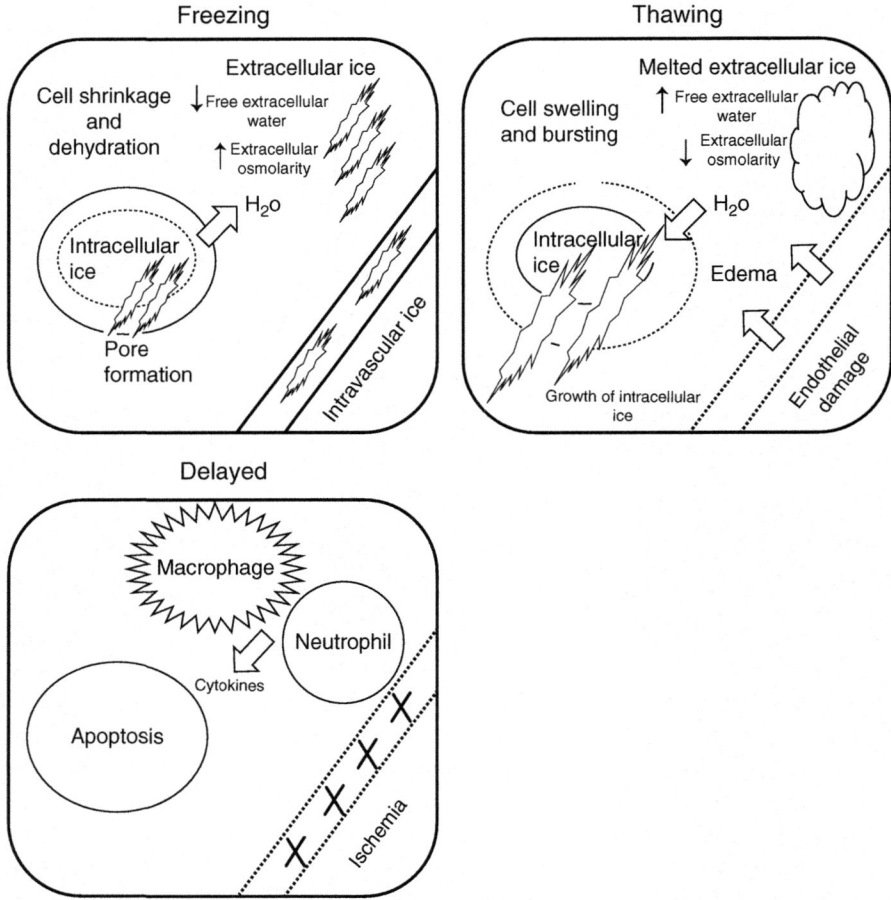

Fig. 3.1 Cryoablation: mechanism of action. During freezing, extracellular ice formation results in sequestration of free extracellular water, increasing the osmolarity of the extracellular space. This leads to cellular dehydration and cell shrinkage. Intracellular ice formation results in disruption of organelle and plasma membranes, impairing cellular function. During thawing, extracellular ice melts before intracellular ice, creating an osmotic fluid shift of water into damaged cells, causing swelling and bursting. Growth of intracellular ice crystals can continue during thawing, exacerbating cellular damage. Damage to the vascular endothelium results in tissue edema. Delayed cellular damage occurs due to the initiation of apoptosis by the cold-induced cellular injury. Thrombosis of blood vessels causes tissue ischemia, hindering repair. Inflammatory cells, including macrophages and neutrophils, remove damaged cells and clear cellular debris

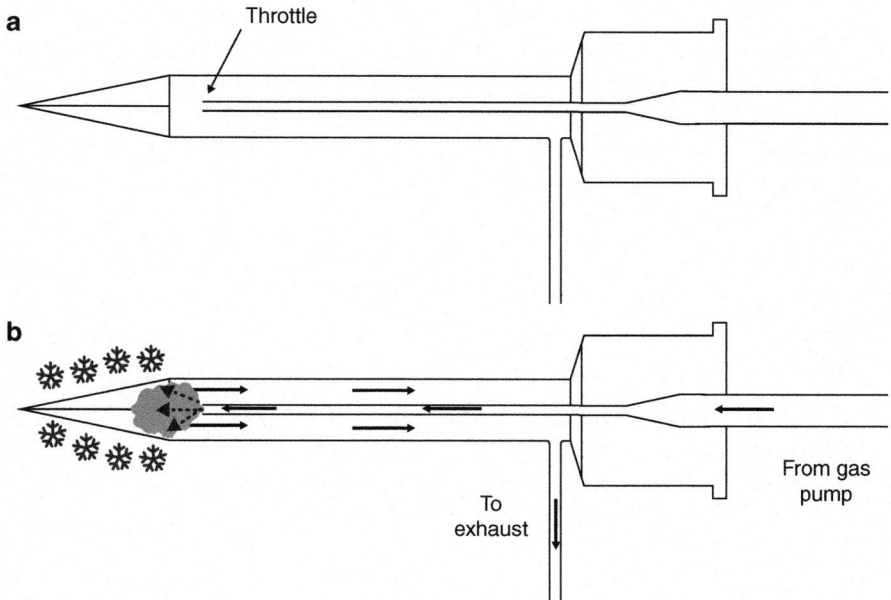

Fig. 3.2 Cryoprobe design. (**a**) A cryoprobe is simply a closed-loop, high-pressure gas-expansion system. (**b**) When the high-pressure room-temperature gas (typically argon) reaches the distal aspect of the cryoprobe, the gas is forced through a narrow opening (throttle). Within the tip of the needle, the argon expands rapidly to atmospheric pressure, causing a marked decrease in the temperature of the gas that is rapidly transferred by convection and conduction to the metallic walls of the cryoprobe. The depressurized gas is vented back out of the hub of the needle

Equipment

Components

- A basic cryoablation system consists of two components: a cryoprobe and a cryoablation system.
- The cryoprobe is essentially a closed-loop, high-pressure gas-expansion system (Fig. 3.2). Temperature change at the tip of the cryoprobe takes place by means of the Joule-Thompson effect, whereby rapid, adiabatic expansion of a gas results in a change in the temperature of the gas [6] that is rapidly transferred to the metallic walls of the cryoprobe.
- To cool the cryoprobe and freeze the tissue, the cryoablation system circulates argon through the cryoprobe, which exhibits Joule-Thompson cooling when quickly expanded within the cryoprobe. To heat the cryoprobe and thaw the tissue, the cryoablation system circulates helium through the cryoprobe, which exhibits Joule-Thompson heating when quickly expanded within the cryoprobe.
- The depressurized gas is vented back out of the hub of the needle through the cryoablation system to the atmosphere.

- Cryoprobes are often insulated along the shaft away from the tip to focus ablation at the tip of the cryoprobe and to minimize nontarget ablation along the shaft.
- The size of the cryoablation zone ("ice ball") can be tailored to the lesion being treated by selecting cryoprobes of various lengths and diameters. Cryoprobe sizes range from 1 to 3 mm, with larger gauge probes yielding greater transaxial-sized cryoablation zones.

Cost

- Cryoablation systems cost approximately $50,000–60,000.
- Cryoprobes cost approximately $1,000–1,200 each.
- For each cryoablation case, cryogen costs (argon and helium) can range from $200 to $500.

Advantages

- The primary advantage of cryoablation over other thermal ablation techniques is the ability to easily monitor the ablation zone during the procedure under real-time radiologic imaging (Fig. 3.3). During freezing, the water of the tissue undergoes a phase transition from liquid to solid, forming an ice ball, which is visible under ultrasound [7], computed tomography [8], and magnetic resonance imaging guidance [9].
- Because the cooling of tissues and nerves provides an anesthetic effect, cryoablation tends to be less painful than heat-based thermal ablation techniques such as microwave or radiofrequency ablation. As such, it typically does not require general anesthesia and is performed in the outpatient setting with moderate sedation.
- Because the cooling mechanism is primarily mechanical rather than electronic, operation of cryoablation devices typically does not cause interference with computed tomography or magnetic resonance imaging machines.
- Each cryoprobe acts independently of others, allowing multiple probes to be used simultaneously to ablate a zone, which conforms to the tumor being treated.
- Cryoablation may be less destructive to structural components of tissue than heat-based thermal ablation, preserving the integrity of basement membrane [10].
- Following cryoablation, tumor proteins remain in situ, whereas coagulative denaturation of proteins occurs with heat-based thermal ablation. The presence of nonviable tumor antigens may potentiate humoral [11] and cell-mediated [12] immune responses, which may enhance the tumoricidal effect of cryoablation.

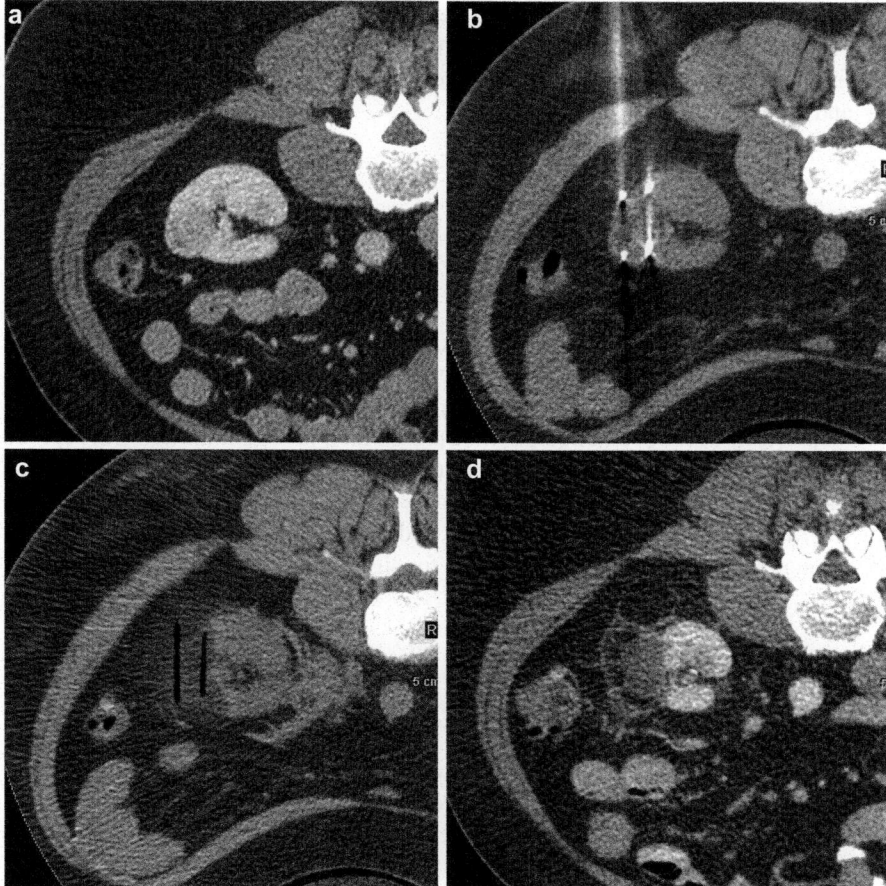

Fig. 3.3 A 47-year-old with renal-cell cancer of the left kidney. The patient was deemed a poor surgical candidate due to morbid obesity and sleep apnea. (**a**) Contrast-enhanced CT scan demonstrates an enhancing tumor in the midzone of the left kidney. Biopsy confirmed clear-cell renal-cell carcinoma. (**b**) Two 2.4-mm cryoprobes are placed in the tumor. (**c**) Following cryoablation and removal of the cryoprobe, a low-attenuation "ice ball" encompasses the lesion and gas tracts are seen in place of the needles. (**d**) Contrast-enhanced CT scans 6 months after cryoablation demonstrates nonenhancement of the tumor and ablation zone, and shrinkage of the residual mass

Disadvantages

- The robust inflammatory response following cryoablation can lead to a systemic inflammatory response syndrome termed cryoshock [13, 14]. This constellation of findings, which can include hypotension, respiratory compromise, multiorgan failure, and disseminated intravascular coagulation, is mediated by cytokine production [15], and has been seen with large volume liver cryoablation.
- Because cryoablation does not use heat, cautery effects and coagulation of injured vessels do not occur, and bleeding complications can be exacerbated.

- Frozen tissues are more brittle than heated tissues, and excessive torque or displacement of cryoprobes while in the tissue can result in organ fracture [16].
- Cryoablation also requires purchase and storage of sufficient quantities of argon and helium gas.

Future of Cryoablation

- Development of cryoablation systems, which do not require rare noble gases. Rapid expansion of common gases like nitrogen in a cryoprobe results in a phase transition from gas to liquid, which can block gas circulation through the needle (vapor lock). However, circulation of pressurized nitrogen through a cryoprobe near its critical point (which refers to the point where there is no distinct phase transition between liquid and gas) can avoid the vapor lock limitation. In this way, circulating gas can be recycled, and large amounts of gases are not lost through venting, creating the potential for significant cost and space savings.

Key Points
- Cryoablation devices create rapid cooling of the cryoprobe via the Joule-Thompson expansion of argon.
- The cold-induced tumor injury sustained through image-guided cryoablation is affected by four factors: cooling rate, target temperature, time at target temperature, and thawing rate.
- The major advantage of cryoablation over other thermal ablative modalities is the ability to directly visualize the ablation zone "ice ball" under radiologic (MR, CT, U/S) guidance.

References

1. Goldberg SN, Grassi CJ, Cardella JF, et al. Image-guided tumor ablation: standardization of terminology and reporting criteria. J Vasc Interv Radiol. 2009;20(7 Suppl):S377–90.
2. Mazur P. Freezing of living cells: mechanisms and implications. Am J Physiol. 1984;247(3 Pt 1): C125–42.
3. Bryant G. DSC measurement of cell suspensions during successive freezing runs: implications for the mechanisms of intracellular ice formation. Cryobiology. 1995;32(2):114–28.
4. Gage AA, Baust J. Mechanisms of tissue injury in cryosurgery. Cryobiology. 1998;37(3): 171–86.
5. Baust JG, Gage AA. The molecular basis of cryosurgery. BJU Int. 2005;95(9):1187–91.
6. O'Rourke AP, Haemmerich D, Prakash P, Converse MC, Mahvi DM, Webster JG. Current status of liver tumor ablation devices. Expert Rev Med Devices. 2007;4(4):523–37.

7. Silverman SG, Tuncali K, Adams DF, Nawfel RD, Zou KH, Judy PF. CT fluoroscopy-guided abdominal interventions: techniques, results, and radiation exposure. Radiology. 1999;212(3):673–81.
8. Tacke J, Speetzen R, Heschel I, Hunter DW, Rau G, Günther RW. Imaging of interstitial cryotherapy – an in vitro comparison of ultrasound, computed tomography, and magnetic resonance imaging. Cryobiology. 1999;38(3):250–9.
9. Tuncali K, Morrison PR, Tatli S, Silverman SG. MRI-guided percutaneous cryoablation of renal tumors: use of external manual displacement of adjacent bowel loops. Eur J Radiol. 2006; 59(2):198–202.
10. Evonich 3rd RF, Nori DM, Haines DE. A randomized trial comparing effects of radiofrequency and cryoablation on the structural integrity of esophageal tissue. J Interv Card Electrophysiol. 2007;19(2):77–83.
11. Ablin RJ, Soanes WA, Gonder MJ. Elution of in vivo bound antiprostatic epithelial antibodies following multiple cryotherapy of carcinoma of prostate. Urology. 1973;2(3):276–9.
12. den Brok MH, Sutmuller RP, Nierkens S, et al. Efficient loading of dendritic cells following cryo and radiofrequency ablation in combination with immune modulation induces antitumour immunity. Br J Cancer. 2006;95(7):896–905.
13. Chapman WC, Debelak JP, Blackwell TS, et al. Hepatic cryoablation-induced acute lung injury: pulmonary hemodynamic and permeability effects in a sheep model. Arch Surg. 2000;135(6):667–72; discussion 72–3.
14. Washington K, Debelak JP, Gobbell C, et al. Hepatic cryoablation-induced acute lung injury: histopathologic findings. J Surg Res. 2001;95(1):1–7.
15. Seifert JK, Stewart GJ, Hewitt PM, Bolton EJ, Junginger T, Morris DL. Interleukin-6 and tumor necrosis factor-alpha levels following hepatic cryotherapy: association with volume and duration of freezing. World J Surg. 1999;23(10):1019–26.
16. Hruby G, Edelstein A, Karpf J, et al. Risk factors associated with renal parenchymal fracture during laparoscopic cryoablation. BJU Int. 2008;102(6):723–6.

Chapter 4
Overview of Thermal Ablation Devices: Microwave

Jeffrey A. Klein, Fred T. Lee Jr., J. Louis Hinshaw, Meghan G. Lubner, and Chris L. Brace

Mechanism of Action

Tissue Heating

- Microwave ablation utilizes dielectric hysteresis to produce heat within tissue.
- Dielectric hysteresis occurs when polar molecules in tissue (primarily H_2O) are forced to continuously realign with an applied, oscillating electromagnetic field.
- The polar molecules will realign billions of times per second, thus increasing their kinetic energy and temperature by friction.
- Tissues with a high percentage of water (as in solid organs and tumors) are most conducive to this type of heating and readily absorb microwave energy.
- Tissue destruction, via coagulation, occurs when tissues are heated to a lethal temperature by the applied electromagnetic frequency of either 915 MHz or 2.45 GHz, which are the only ISM (industrial, scientific, and medical) approved frequencies.

J.A. Klein, M.D. • F.T. Lee Jr., M.D. (✉) • J.L. Hinshaw, M.D. • M.G. Lubner, M.D.
Department of Radiology, University of Wisconsin, School of Medicine and Public Health,
E3/311 Clinical Science Center, 600 Highland Avenue, Madison, WI 53792-3252, USA
e-mail: jklein@uwhealth.org; flee@uwhealth.org

C.L. Brace, Ph.D.
Department of Radiology, University of Wisconsin, School of Medicine
and Public Health, E3/311 Clinical Science Center, 600 Highland Avenue,
Madison, WI 53792-3252, USA
e-mail: cbrace@uwhealth.org

T. Clark, T. Sabharwal (eds.), *Interventional Radiology Techniques in Ablation*, 21
Techniques in Interventional Radiology,
DOI 10.1007/978-0-85729-094-6_4, © Springer-Verlag London 2013

Equipment

Components of a Microwave System

- The basic microwave system consists of three components: a generator, a power distribution system, and an interstitial antenna(s) (Fig. 4.1).
- Microwave ablation generators utilize one of two basic power sources: a magnetron or solid-state amplifier. The generators have different performance characteristics (e.g., differences in output power and efficiency), but both ultimately produce the electromagnetic energy that is transmitted from the generator to the target tissue.
- The power distribution system is most commonly composed of coaxial cables, because of their flexibility, compact size, and propagation characteristics.
- The size and flexibility of the coaxial cables is currently limited by a balance between the ability to transmit higher energy to the antenna while avoiding the inherent heating of the cable itself – as the cable diameter decreases, power loss and cable heating increase.
- Antennas come in varying sizes and geometries, but are generally straight, needle-like applicators that are positioned in the target tissue via a percutaneous, laparoscopic, or open surgical approach.
- Since antennas are generally constructed from coaxial cables, the same limitation of balancing the antenna diameter while avoiding unwanted heating of the shaft applies.
- To increase power handling of smaller diameter antennas, reduce shaft heating, and eliminate nontarget ablation along the insertion tract, cooling jackets and antenna-cooling systems are generally necessary.
- Circulation of chilled saline is currently the most commonly utilized method for cooling the antenna shaft, thus enabling the delivery of higher powers for longer periods of time.
- Circulating compressed carbon dioxide along both the coaxial cables and the antenna shaft is another method utilized. This method allows for a higher cooling capacity, resulting in the ability to use higher power generators and smaller antenna diameters, which result in shorter ablation times and a less-invasive approach.

Cost

- The cost of microwave generators is generally higher than radiofrequency (RF) generators.
- The cost of microwave antennas varies by company.

Fig. 4.1 Certus 140–
2.45 GHz, 140 W Ablation
System by NeuWave
Medical, Inc. (Madison, WI)

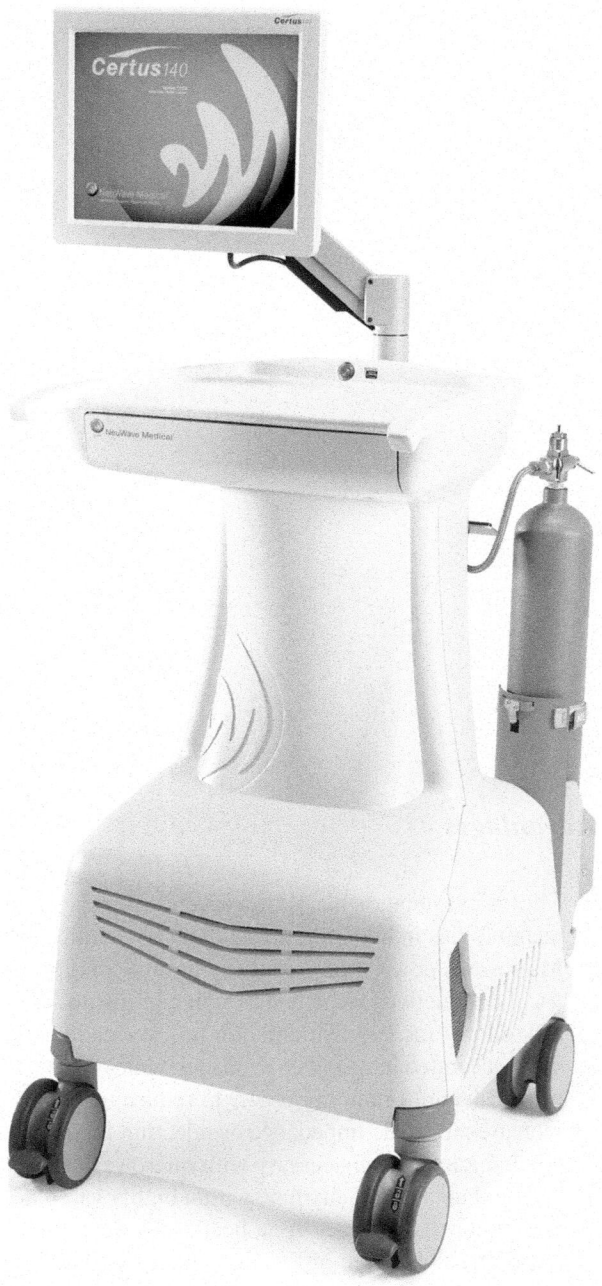

Fig. 4.1 (continued)

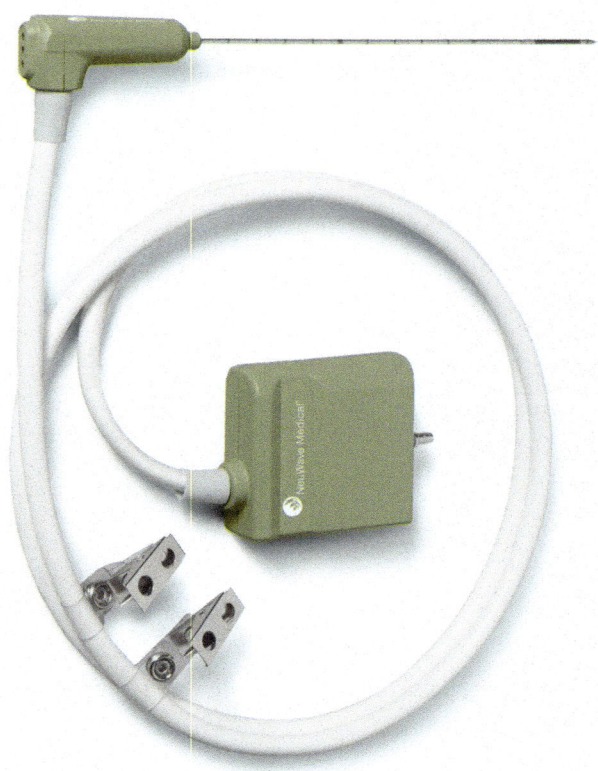

Advantages

- Microwave ablation has shown several advantages over other heat-based ablation technologies in both preclinical and early clinical trials.
- Microwave power can propagate through all types of tissues, regardless of electrical conductivity, which stands in contrast to RF electrical current. This property allows for efficient ablation in low-conductivity (high-impedance) tissues, such as aerated lung and charred, dessicated tissue, a major limitation in RF ablation. Pulsing or ramping power to reduce temperature elevation and subsequent increases in tissue impedance or injecting fluids into the target tissue to increase conductivity are unnecessary with microwave ablation.
- Thermal ablation of any type within highly vascularized tissues, such as the liver and kidney, is hindered by a heat-sink effect, which limits both the achievable temperature and size of the ablation zone. Microwave ablation has been shown to be less susceptible to vascular cooling by the heat-sink effect, resulting in faster heating and higher achievable temperatures. This characteristic results in several advantages compared to RF ablation:
  - Increased ablation zone size, allowing for the successful treatment of larger tumors (>3 cm) (Fig. 4.2).

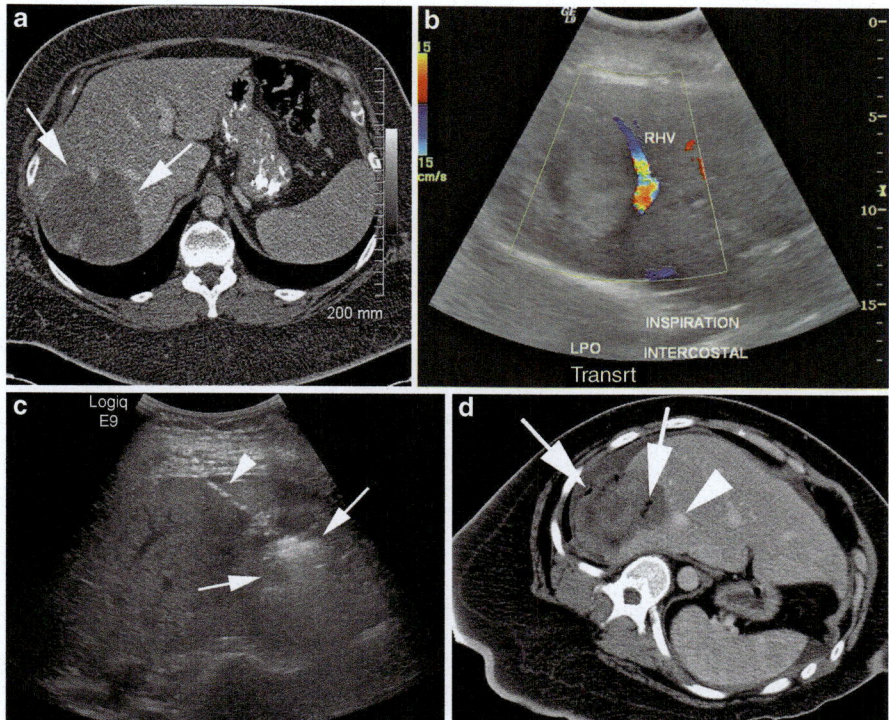

Fig. 4.2 A 39-year-old female with a large symptomatic hepatic hemangioma. (**a**) Pretreatment CT image demonstrates an 8.3 × 8.7 cm hemangioma (*arrows*). (**b**) Pretreatment ultrasound demonstrates the lesions in proximity to the right hepatic vein (RHV). (**c**) Three Certus 140, 15-cm 17-gauge antennas were placed into the lesion in a linear array. The central antenna was powered at 140 W for 5 min. Subsequently, all three antennas were powered at 65 W for 10 min. Grayscale ultrasound image during the initial ablation with the single antenna (*arrowhead*) demonstrates the development of a large ablation zone (*arrows*). (**d**) Posttreatment CT image demonstrates complete ablation of the hemangioma (note macroscopic gas in the periphery of the mass (*arrows*)) with preserved patency of the adjacent right hepatic vein (*arrowhead*). Total ablation time was 15 min with an ablation zone of 9.2×7.7×6.6 cm

- More effective ablation in close proximity to large vessels (>3 mm in diameter), increasing the spectrum of patients that can be treated with ablation.
- Decreased ablation time, translating to more efficient use of equipment and personnel, decrease in time a patient requires sedation or general anesthesia, and allowing for an increase in the number of tumors that can reasonably be treated during a single ablation session (Fig. 4.3).

- Microwaves do not rely on an electrical circuit to transmit energy, thus eliminating the requirement to use a ground pad or a second interstitial applicator to complete an electrical circuit.
- Microwave ablation supports multiple applicator ablations to increase ablation zone size and decrease procedure time. Unlike RF ablation, the antennas can all

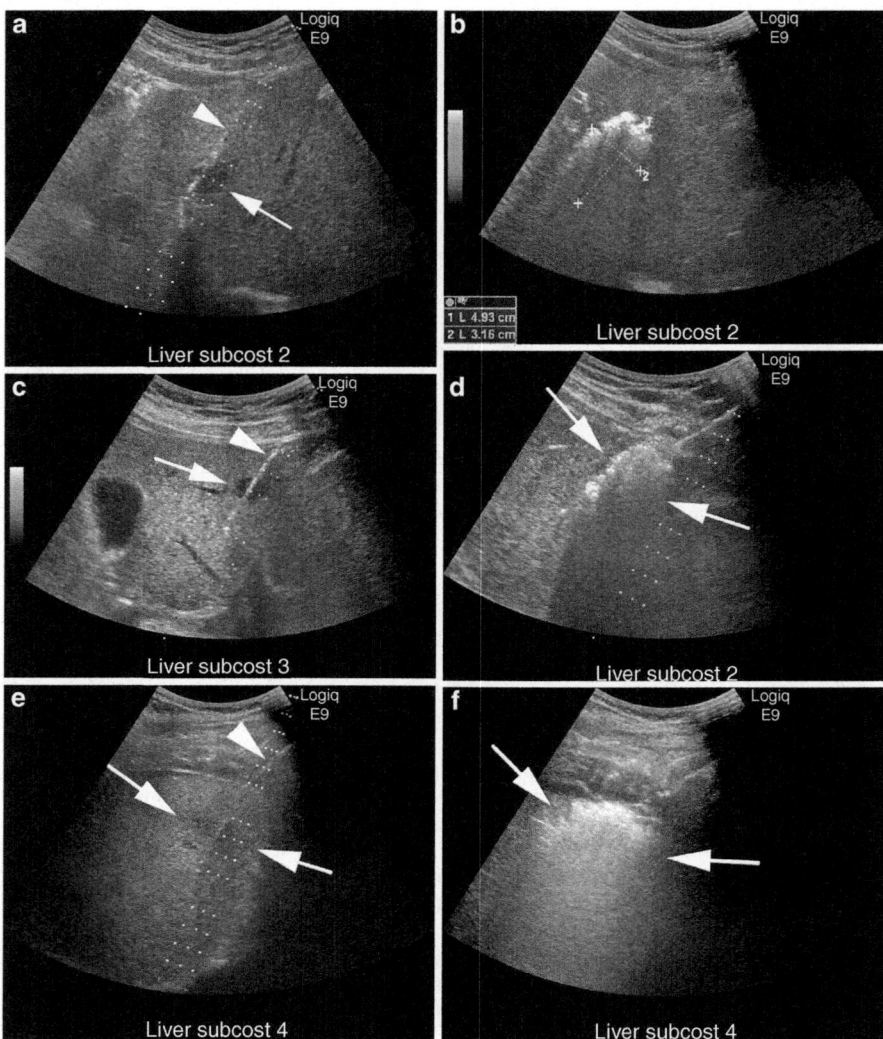

Fig. 4.3 A 65-year-old male with four hepatic leiomyosarcoma metastatic lesions, all of which were treated with microwave ablation (three shown here). (**a**) A single antenna (*arrowhead*) was eccentrically positioned within a 1.7-cm metastasis in segment IVa (*arrow*) and treated at 140 W for 6 min. (**b**) This resulted in a large ablation zone (calipers) and a technically successful ablation. (**c**) Similarly, a single antenna (*arrowhead*) was more centrally positioned in a 1.2-cm metastasis in segment IVb (*arrow*). (**d**) Because of the improved positioning, this metastasis could be fully ablated (*arrows*) in only 4 min at 140 W. (**e**) A larger, 3.1-cm metastasis in segment VIII (*arrows*) required placement of two antennas, one of which is seen (*arrowhead*). (**f**) The antenna were powered at 95 W for 5 min, resulting in a large ablation zone that fully encompassed the metastasis (*arrows*). All lesions were treated during a single ablation session. (**g–i**) Posttreatment CT demonstrated a technically successful ablation for all metastasis (*arrows*)

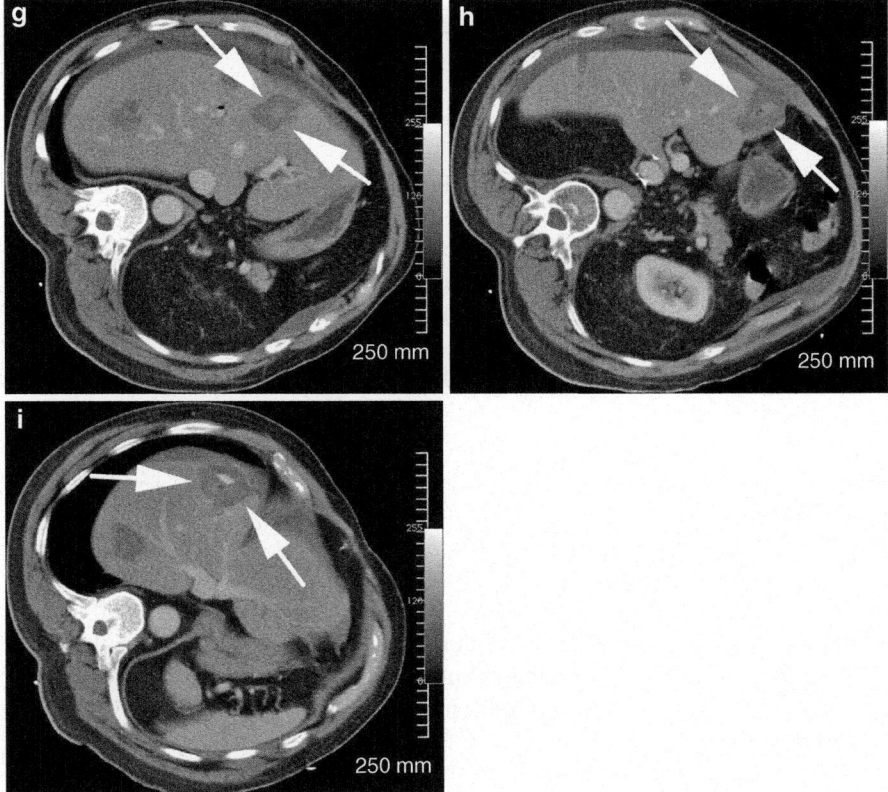

Fig. 4.3 (continued)

be activated simultaneously, eliminating the need to switch between applicators and thus improving the efficiency and synergy of the heating.

Disadvantages

- Microwave energy is inherently more difficult to generate and deliver to the tissue compared to RF due to the complexity of the generators and the requirement to deliver energy via coaxial cables. Coaxial cables are larger in diameter, stiffer, and more prone to heating than the simple wires used in current RF systems.
- Though the capability of delivering larger amounts of energy, obtaining higher temperatures, creating larger ablation zones, and decreasing ablation time exists for microwave technology, the technical hurdles to control the distribution of this power safely must be overcome.
- Larger and faster ablation zones may increase the potential for heating nontargeted structures, with resultant collateral damage.
- The clinical data are currently less robust for microwave than for RF ablation.

Future of Microwave Ablation

- As microwave ablation technology progresses, foreseeable advancements include:

  - Use of constructive and destructive interference (wave propagation) to achieve more customizable ablation zones.
  - Utilization of a broadened frequency spectrum to improve ablation efficiency and, again, achieve more customizable ablation zones.
  - Development of smaller gauge antenna to further decrease the invasiveness of ablation treatment.
  - Miniaturization and modification of equipment to accommodate other access routes (i.e. endoscopic).

Key Points
- Microwave ablation utilizes dielectric hysteresis to produce heat, which occurs when polar molecules are forced to continuously realign with an oscillating electromagnetic field.
- Advantages of microwave ablation over other heat-based technologies include: efficient ablation in low conductivity tissues, reduced susceptibility to the heat-sink effect, faster heating, higher achievable temperatures, and larger ablation zones.

Suggested Reading

Brace CL. Microwave ablation technology: what every user should know. Curr Probl Diagn Radiol. 2009a;38:61–7.

Brace CL. Radiofrequency and microwave ablation of the liver, lung, kidney, and bone: what are the differences? Curr Probl Diagn Radiol. 2009b;38:135–43.

Lubner MG, Brace CL, Hinshaw JL, Lee Jr FT. Microwave tumor ablation: mechanism of action, clinical results, and devices. J Vasc Interv Radiol. 2010;21:S192–203.

Chapter 5
Overview of Thermal Ablation Devices: HIFU, Laser Interstitial, Chemical Ablation

Julien Garnon, Georgia Tsoumakidou, Iulian Enescu, Xavier Buy, and Afshin Gangi

High-Intensity Focused Ultrasound (HIFU) Ablation

Introduction

HIFU is a noninvasive ablation technique, which uses the property of ultrasounds (US) to propagate harmlessly energy through human tissues. HIFU focuses high-intensity US waves into a target area, thus generating focal deposition of high energy that leads to cellular death in living tissues.

History of HIFU

- Biological effects of HIFU were first reported in 1927 by Wood et al. [1].
- The possibility that this technique may produce highly localized biological effects was introduced in the early 1940s [2].
- First clinical applications of HIFU were performed in the 1950s to produce focal lesions in the brains of animals and then in the brains of patients suffering from Parkinson's disease [3].

J. Garnon, M.D. (✉) • G. Tsoumakidou, M.D. • I. Enescu, M.D.
X. Buy, M.D. • A. Gangi, M.D., Ph.D.
Department of Interventional Radiology, University Hospital of Strasbourg, 1, place de l'Hopital, BP 426, 67091 Strasbourg, France
e-mail: julien.garnon@chru-strasbourg.fr; xavier.buy@chru-strasbourg.fr; gangi@rad6.u-strasbg.fr

T. Clark, T. Sabharwal (eds.), *Interventional Radiology Techniques in Ablation*, Techniques in Interventional Radiology,
DOI 10.1007/978-0-85729-094-6_5, © Springer-Verlag London 2013

- Although it looked effective, clinical use of HIFU for the treatment of Parkinson's disease stayed confidential because of the complexity and the risks of the procedure, and the concomitant development of L-Dopa treatment.
- During the next 30 years, publications concerning HIFU looked at the properties of focused US in normal tissues.
- Regain of interest for HIFU ablation in clinical application occurred in the 1990s with the improvement of imaging. Technological innovations such as ultrasonography and magnetic resonance imaging made it possible to visualize precisely the lesions to target and thus to use HIFU for focal oncological treatment [4].

Principles of HIFU

- US is a cyclic sound pressure with a frequency above the human hearing range (above 20,000 Hz).
- The intensity of US is proportional to sonic pressure and is measured in W/cm [5]. Basically, the higher the pressure is, the more energy the US wave will carry.
- Diagnostic ultrasonography is one of the major applications of US, with frequencies ranging between 1 and 20 MHz.
- US beam carries a certain quantity of energy, which propagates and interacts with living tissues.
- Diagnostic US delivers acoustic intensities around 100 mW/cm^2 (720 mW/cm^2 maximum), which have no side effects on human organs.
- HIFU relies on the same principle as conventional US. US waves are used to propagate energy through the human body without damaging the organs.
- By focusing high-intensity US beams, acoustic intensity in the focused area is several orders greater (>10 W/cm^2) than with conventional US [6]. This results in a focal deposition of high energy, which produces coagulation necrosis in living tissues (Fig. 5.1).

Mechanisms of HIFU Ablation

Tissue ablation results of two main effects of HIFU: the thermal effect and the mechanical effects [7, 8].

Thermal Effect

- Thermal toxicity depends on exposure time and temperature elevation.
- In biological tissues, coagulation necrosis occurs if the local temperature rises above the threshold of 56°C during at least 1 s.

Fig. 5.1 HIFU ablation: the HIFU beam goes through the skin and the tissues and creates a cigar-shaped lesion at the focus

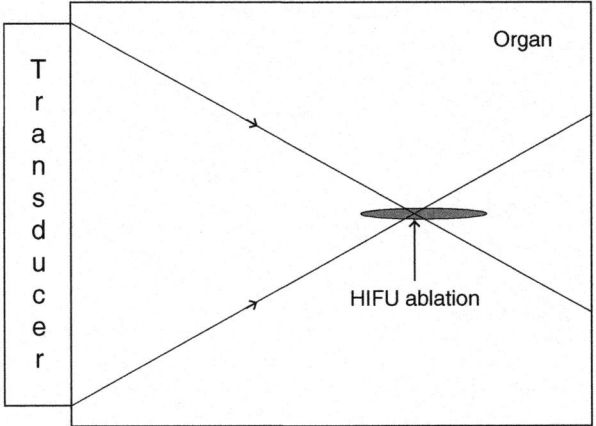

- Whether it is with diagnostic or therapeutic US, absorption of US waves in human tissues causes molecular agitation and thus frictional heat.
- With conventional US, molecular agitation is minimal.
- With HIFU, absorption of high-intensity US waves at the focus generates a quick elevation of temperature (>60°C), which exceeds the rate of vascular perfusion cooling of the tissues, thus leading to instantaneous and irreversible cell death via coagulation necrosis.

Mechanical Effects

Mechanical effects only appear with high-intensity US and include cavitation and radiation force.

Cavitation

- Cavitation is a complex and unpredictable mechanism, which corresponds to the formation of gas cavity in a tissue.
- When a high-intensity US beam propagates through a medium, it causes vibration and subjects the molecular structure to alternating compression and expansion. This phenomenon leads to cavitation.
- There are two types of cavitation: stable (or noninertial) cavitation and unstable (or inertial) cavitation:

- Stable cavitation corresponds to the stable oscillation of the size of the bubbles. Rapid movement of the bubbles produces acoustic microstreaming, which creates high shear forces that may damage cell membranes.
- Unstable cavitation is the expanding oscillation of the size of the bubbles, which leads finally to disintegration of the gas cavity in a violent collapse. Rupture of the bubbles produces both high mechanical stress and temperatures, which contribute to cellular death.

Radiation Force

- Radiation force occurs when high-intensity US waves are absorbed or reflected by a free fluid medium.
- Transfer of energy from the US field creates movement of the fluid (acoustic streaming), which produces shear stress and may induce cell apoptosis.

HIFU Systems

Focus of High-Intensity US Waves

- First generation of HIFU devices used concave-shaped transducers or flat transducers combined with an acoustic lens to focus the US beams.
- Drawbacks of these systems were the lack of versatility (concave-shaped transducers) and attenuation of the US beam (systems with the acoustic lens).
- Current HIFU systems use the phased array technology to focus US waves into a tight area. Each component of the transducer receives its own modifiable electronic signal. This technique allows to steer and to focus the US beams, which enables to move the focus in almost any direction [6].
- The destruction induced by a single exposure has an ellipsoidal shape with a size of about 1.5 mm in width and 15 mm in length ("cigar" shape). This size may vary from a few millimeters depending on the parameters of the transducer.
- In clinical practice, tumor usually measures more than 1 cm. Several overlapping shots have to be performed to ablate the whole lesion with safety margins and without leaving any residual viable tissue (Fig. 5.2).
- The need to repeat the shots makes the intervention time-consuming (several hours for most of the tumors treated in clinical practice). It is currently one of the main limitations of HIFU ablation.

Transducers

There are two main categories of transducers: the extracorporeal and the transrectal systems. Another type of device, the interstitial transducer, is being developed for the ablation of esophageal and biliary lesions.

Fig. 5.2 HIFU ablation: overlapping shots are necessary to ablate the tumor without leaving any viable tissue

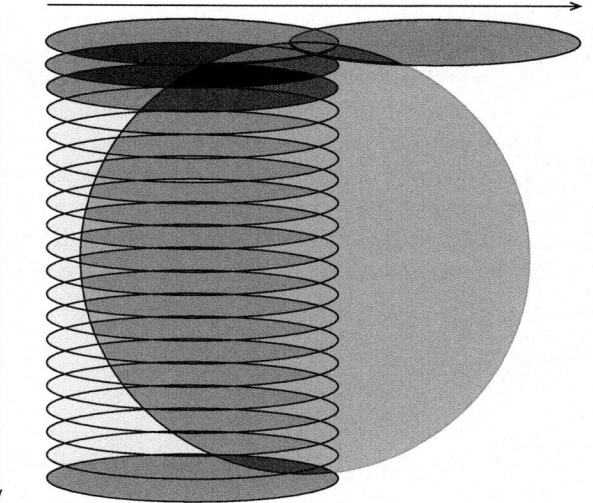

Extracorporeal Devices

- Extracorporeal devices are used to treat various benign and malignant conditions in superficial organs (thyroid, breast) or more deep-seated structures such as the abdominal and pelvic organs.
- Because there is usually a long distance between the transducer and the targeted organ, these devices usually work with high power and low frequencies (around 1 MHz) to minimize the attenuation of US waves [8].
- Ablation with extracorporeal systems may be guided by US or magnetic resonance imaging (MRI).

Transrectal Devices

- Transrectal devices are indicated for the treatment of benign and malignant pathologies of the prostate.
- As the transducer lies close to the target volume, there are less sonic attenuation and loss of power during the propagation of US waves than with extracorporeal devices. Transrectal systems thus work with low power and high frequencies (around 8 MHz) to maximize the precision of the focal ablation [9].
- Transrectal HIFU is monitored by US guidance.

Image Guidance

- Imaging has two major goals in HIFU ablation: to visualize precisely the zone to be ablated (guidance of HIFU) and to evaluate local temperature during the ablative phase (monitoring of HIFU).
- Both US-guided HIFU and MRI-guided HIFU devices exist, each system having its advantages and drawbacks.

US-Guided HIFU

- Guidance of HIFU: ultrasonography shares the same entry point and the same acoustic window as HIFU. Adequate imaging of the tumor on B-mode US is therefore necessary to perform HIFU ablation. US guidance may be insufficient in case of poor tissue contrast resolution, bone or gas interposition, and deep-seated tumors.
- Monitoring of HIFU: US is not yet able to assess local temperature. During HIFU exposure, the hyperechoic changes on B-mode are secondary to local cavitation and boiling and are not reflecting precisely the zone of coagulation necrosis [6].

MR-Guided HIFU

- Guidance of HIFU: MRI offers high contrast resolution and large fields of view, thereby providing good delineation of tumors in most cases. Spatial resolution and motion artifacts may limit accuracy of MRI in some patients.
- Monitoring of HIFU: changes in water proton resonance frequency are dependent on temperature. MRI thus offers the possibility to evaluate local temperature in the treated tissue (MR thermometry), which is helpful to determine if coagulation necrosis has occurred [10]. However, MR thermometry has some drawbacks: it usually underestimates local temperature, it is insensitive to changes of temperature in fat, and it may be altered by motion artifacts.

Clinical Applications

HIFU Ablation (Focused US Surgery)

- Ablation is currently the major application of HIFU.
- HIFU has been used to treat various benign and malignant conditions such as benign prostatic hyperplasia [11], carcinoma of the prostate [12], hepatocellular carcinoma [13], kidney cancer [14], pancreatic cancer [15], bone metastases [16], breast cancer [17], and uterine fibroids [18].
- The targeted volume must include the tumor and safety margins (5–10 mm). Ill-defined tumors and tumors lying closely (<5 mm) to vital structures should therefore not be treated with HIFU.
- The skin entry point should be shaved and scar free in order not to create an interface for US, which may lead to cavitation and skin burn.
- A clear acoustic window has to be found to target the lesion because air, gas, and bone interfere with the propagation of the US waves.
- These interfaces may cause:

  - US absorption with a risk of undertreatment of the underlying tumor.
  - Local cavitation with a risk of burns in the intervening tissues.

- Anesthesia (conscious sedation or general anesthesia) is necessary in almost all cases to prevent pain and to ensure patient's immobilization during ablation.

- The power of treatment depends of the location (organ, depth) of the tumor.
- Power is increased stepwise under the control of imaging (US and MRI) and real-time temperature (MRI only).
- Postablation necrosis is evaluated with contrast-enhanced examination (CT or MRI).

Other Applications

- Targeted drug delivery: selective insonation of preloaded microbubbles or nanoparticles increases the concentration of drugs at the focus and decreases the systemic toxicity of these agents.
- Enhancement of immune response: according to some reports, HIFU may activate a systemic host tumor – specific immune response [19].
- Vessel occlusion: in experimental studies, HIFU proved to be effective to interrupt blood flow in small vessels [20].

Conclusion

HIFU is currently the only complete noninvasive ablation technique with interventional oncology as the main field of indications. Although it looks promising, HIFU therapy still have some limitations, like duration of intervention, and must be further evaluated. Technological innovations will contribute to improve this technology.

Interstitial Laser Ablation

Introduction

Interstitial laser ablation consists of percutaneous insertion of one (or several) optical fiber(s) inside a tumor. Laser then acts as a point heat source, which destructs cells by direct heating.

Characteristics of the Laser System

- Interstitial laser ablation uses infrared wavelengths between 700 and 1,200 nm [21].
- Two types of devices can be used in clinical practice:
    - The neodymium yttrium aluminum garnet (Nd:YAG) laser, which have a precise wavelength of 1,064 nm
    - The diode lasers, which have variable wavelengths (usually between 800 and 1,000 nm)

- The optical fiber is 400–600 μm in size and can be up to 10 m in length. It can pass through an 18-gauge needle.
- The fiber is not interacting with pacemakers and metallic structures, and is MRI-compatible.
- Several optical fibers can be connected to the laser generator in the same time.

Mechanisms of Action

- When laser energy is delivered at the tip of the optical fiber, it scatters within tissues.
- This scattering converts laser energy into heat, which causes coagulation necrosis.
- Destruction occurs from the center to the periphery.
- The size of the ablation zone depends on:

  – The size of the optical fiber
  – The laser wavelength
  – The thermal and optical properties of the tissue
  – The power and duration of laser application:

$$Energy\ delivered\ (Joules) = Power\ (Watts) \times Time\ (Seconds)$$

- For example, with a laser wavelength of 800 nm and a power of 2 W during 10 min, the energy delivered in the tissue is about 1,200 J and the diameter of coagulation is 15 mm maximum. Delivering more than 1,200 J with the same needle position is not useful as it does not increase the size of coagulation.
- Internally cooled laser can be used to avoid carbonization around the fiber tip and to increase the size of ablation [22].

Clinical Indications

- Interstitial laser ablation has been used in various indications such as percutaneous ablation of breast cancers, pancreatic cancers, lymph nodes, and liver metastases [23]. Depending on the size of the lesions, several optical fibers and/or internally cooled systems can be used to obtain large ablation areas.
- Curative treatment of osteoid osteoma is a very good indication of laser ablation [24].

Procedure

- Interstitial laser ablation requires conscious sedation, spinal anesthesia, or general anesthesia depending on the localization and the type of lesion.

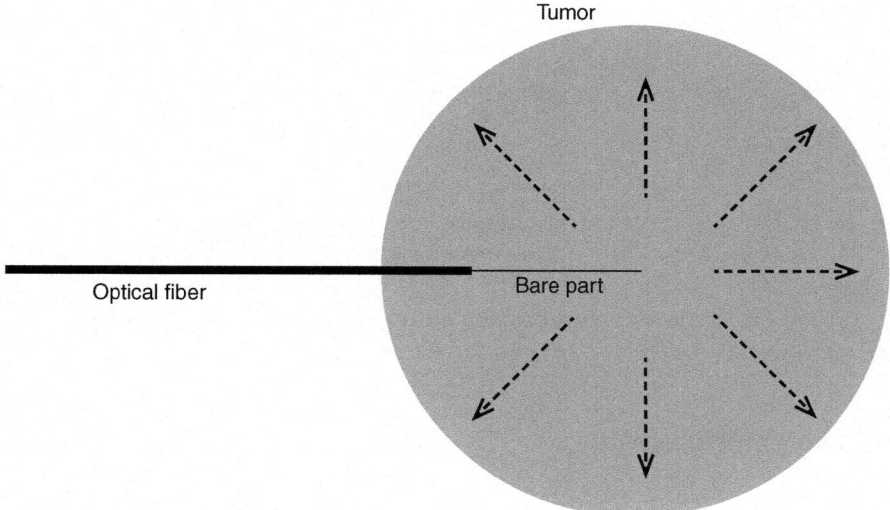

Fig. 5.3 Laser ablation: the bare tip of the optical fiber has to be positioned in the center of the lesion. Ablation occurs from the center to the periphery

- An 18-gauge needle is positioned into the tumor under image guidance. When treating osteoid osteoma, a bony trocar is used to pass through the cortical bone.
- The optical fiber is introduced coaxially through the needle. The tip of the bare fiber should be located at the center of the lesion (Fig. 5.3).
- Power and duration of ablation depends on the size and the localization of the tumor.

Conclusion

Interstitial laser ablation is an easily available technique since it is used in other specialities (like gastro-enterology to treat lesions in esophagus or colon). It allows to produce small predictable volume of necrosis and is therefore one of the best techniques to treat small tumors like osteoid osteoma.

Chemical Ablation

Introduction

Chemical ablation relies on the percutaneous injection of a chemical agent to induce cell death.

Chemical Agents

- Two main chemical agents are used in clinical practice:
  - Ethanol
  - Acetic acid
- Mechanisms of action are the same for both agents (see below).
- Acetic acid diffuses better than ethanol and has the ability to go through tumor septa [25].
- Acetic acid produces a bigger area of necrosis than ethanol at equal volume, and may therefore be preferred to treat large tumors.

Mechanisms of Action

Cellular necrosis is secondary to both cellular and vascular effects of the chemical agent.

Cellular Effects

Ethanol and acetic acid cause dehydration of the cytoplasm and denaturation of cellular proteins, followed by fibrous reaction.

Vascular Effects

Ethanol and acetic acid induce necrosis of endothelial cells and platelet aggregation, which lead to vascular thrombosis and ischemia.

Clinical Applications

Tumor Ablation

- Chemical ablation is the cheapest and easiest method for percutaneous ablation of tumors.
- Treatment of hepatocellular carcinoma is the most accepted indication of percutaneous ethanol injection.
- Chemical ablation has been used to treat other malignant conditions such as adrenal tumors [25] and painful bone tumors [26].
- It is also efficient to treat benign thyroid nodules [27].
- The arrival of thermal ablation techniques has reduced the indications of ethanol ablation. However, a combination of ethanol injection and thermal ablation can be interesting in some indications, like ablation of hepatocellular carcinoma [28].

Fig. 5.4 Splanchnic
neurolysis: two 22-gauge
spinal needles are placed
close to the splanchnic nerves
with a posterior approach
under CT guidance. A
mixture of contrast medium
and local anesthetic is
injected to confirm the proper
distribution before ethanol
injection

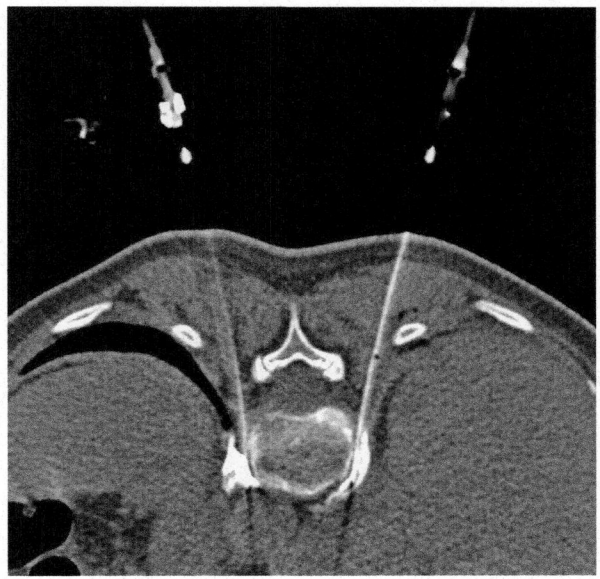

- Chemical ablation is a painful procedure (especially in bone) and usually requires at least conscious sedation.
- The procedure is performed under CT guidance or combined fluoroscopic-US guidance.
- A 22-gauge spinal needle is placed into the tumor, in a non-necrotic part.
- Contrast medium is injected to predict the distribution. If contrast is diffusing beyond the tumor boundaries and approaches critical structures (especially nerves), injection of the chemical agent cannot be performed.
- The volume of injection depends mainly on the size of the lesion and the type of chemical agent. This volume usually ranges between 5 and 25 ml in most cases.
- Needle needs sometimes to be repositioned to cover the whole lesion.

Neurolysis

- Percutaneous ethanol injection is a very effective method to treat pain secondary to the tumorous invasion of a sympathetic plexus [29].
- The site of injection depends on the location of the tumor. For example, epigastric pain related to pancreatic cancer may be relieved by coeliac or splanchnic neurolysis.
- Procedure is performed under local anesthesia.
- CT guidance is the best modality to guide these procedures, but fluoroscopy may be sufficient in some cases.
- A 22-gauge needle is positioned in contact with the involved plexus.
- Contrast medium is injected to confirm the good position of the needle's tip and 5–20 ml of ethanol is administered (Fig. 5.4).
- Relief of pain should happen very quickly after the procedure.

Limitations

* Diffusion of the chemical agent is not predictable, nor controllable.
* Degree of necrosis is highly variable.
* Size of ablation is limited to the treated lesion without safety margins.

Conclusion

Chemical ablation is a fast and cheap procedure, which is very effective in palliative indications. Due to its limitations, chemical ablation should not be used on its own in a curative intent.

References

1. Wood RW, Loomis AL. The physical and biological effects of high frequency sound waves of great intensity. Philos Mag. 1927;4:417.
2. Lynn JG, Zwemer RL, Chick AJ, et al. A new method for the generation and use of focused ultrasound in experimental biology. J Gen Physiol. 1942;26:179–93.
3. Fry WJ, Barnard JW, Fry FJ, et al. Ultrasonically produced localized selective lesions in the central nervous system. Am J Phys Med. 1955;34:413–23.
4. Visioli AG, Rivens IH, ter Haar GR, et al. Preliminary results of a phase I dose escalation clinical trial using focused ultrasound in the treatment of localised tumours. Eur J Ultrasound. 1999;9:11–8.
5. Crocker MJ. Encyclopedia of acoustics. 1st ed. New York: Wiley; 1997. p. 6.
6. Kim YS, Rhim H, Choi MJ, et al. High-intensity focused ultrasound therapy: an overview for radiologists. Korean J Radiol. 2008;9:291–302.
7. Kennedy JE, ter Haar GR, Cranston D. High intensity focused ultrasound: surgery of the future? Br J Radiol. 2003;76:590–9.
8. Zhou YF. High intensity focused ultrasound in clinical tumor ablation. World J Clin Oncol. 2011;2(1):8–27.
9. Haar GT, Coussios C. High intensity focused ultrasound: physical principles and devices. Int J Hyperthermia. 2007;23:89–104.
10. Jolesz FA, McDannold N. Current status and future potential of MRI-guided focused ultrasound surgery. J Magn Reson Imaging. 2008;27:391–9.
11. Sullivan LD, McLoughlin MG, Goldenberg LG, et al. Early experience with high-intensity focused ultrasound for the treatment of benign prostatic hypertrophy. Br J Urol. 1997;79:172–6.
12. Beerlage HP, Thüroff S, Debruyne FM, et al. Transrectal high-intensity focused ultrasound using the Ablatherm device in the treatment of localized prostate carcinoma. Urology. 1999;54:273–7.
13. Li CX, Xu GL, Jiang ZY, et al. Analysis of clinical effect of high-intensity focused ultrasound on liver cancer. World J Gastroenterol. 2004;10:2201–4.
14. Wu F, Wang ZB, Chen WZ, et al. Preliminary experience using high intensity focused ultrasound for the treatment of patients with advanced stage renal malignancy. J Urol. 2003;170: 2237–40.
15. Wu F, Wang ZB, Zhu H, et al. Feasibility of US-guided high-intensity focused ultrasound treatment in patients with advanced pancreatic cancer: initial experience. Radiology. 2005; 236:1034–40.

16. Liberman B, Gianfelice D, Inbar Y, et al. Pain palliation in patients with bone metastases using MR-guided focused ultrasound surgery: a multicenter study. Ann Surg Oncol. 2009;16:140–6.
17. Wu F, Wang ZB, Zhu H, et al. Extracorporeal high intensity focused ultrasound treatment for patients with breast cancer. Breast Cancer Res Treat. 2005;92:51–60.
18. LeBlang SD, Hoctor K, Steinberg FL. Leiomyoma shrinkage after MRI-guided focused ultrasound treatment: report of 80 patients. AJR Am J Roentgenol. 2010;194:274–80.
19. Wu F, Zhou L, Chen WR. Host antitumour immune response to HIFU ablation. Int J Hyperthermia. 2007;23:165–71.
20. Vaezy S, Martin R, Crum L. High intensity focused ultrasound: a method of hemostasis. Echocardiography. 2001;18:309–15.
21. Gangi A, Gasser B, De Unamuno S, et al. New trends in interstitial laser photocoagulation of bones. Semin Musculoskelet Radiol. 1997;1:331–8.
22. Vogl TJ, Mack MG, Roggan A, et al. Internally cooled power laser for MR-guided interstitial laser-induced thermotherapy of liver lesions: initial clinical results. Radiology. 1998;209: 381–5.
23. Amin Z, Donald JJ, Masters A, et al. Hepatic metastases: interstitial laser photocoagulation with real-time US monitoring and dynamic CT evaluation of treatment. Radiology. 1993; 187:339–47.
24. Gangi A, Alizadeh H, Wong L, et al. Osteoid osteoma: percutaneous laser ablation and follow-up in 114 patients. Radiology. 2007;242:293–301.
25. Xiao YY, Tian JL, Li JK, et al. CT-guided percutaneous chemical ablation of adrenal neoplasms. AJR Am J Roentgenol. 2008;190:105–10.
26. Gangi A, Kastler BA, Klinkert A, et al. Injection of alcohol into bone metastases under CT guidance. J Comput Assist Tomogr. 1994;18:932–5.
27. Sung JY, Kim YS, Choi H, et al. Optimum first-line treatment technique for benign cystic thyroid nodules: ethanol ablation or radiofrequency ablation? AJR Am J Roentgenol. 2011; 196:210–4.
28. Azab M, Zaki S, El-Shetey AG, et al. Radiofrequency ablation combined with percutaneous ethanol injection in patients with hepatocellular carcinoma. Arab J Gastroenterol. 2011; 12:113–8.
29. Gangi A, Dietemann JL, Schultz A, et al. Interventional radiologic procedures with CT guidance in cancer pain management. Radiographics. 1996;16:1289–304.

Chapter 6
Overview of Thermal Ablation: Plasma-Mediated Ablation

Konstantinos Katsanos

Terms and Definitions

Plasma-mediated ablation uses bipolar radiofrequency energy to excite the electrolytes in a conductive medium, such as saline solution, creating a precisely focused plasma ion field. The high-energy ionized plasma breaks down intramolecular bonds and produces local decompression by cavitating or dissolving soft tissue at relatively low temperatures. In the literature, it is otherwise referred to as radiofrequency ionization, plasma-radiofrequency or plasma-RF ablation, or controlled ablation or cold ablation. Alternatively, the term coblation has been coined, that is actually a registered trademark of ArthroCare, US, pioneer of plasma-mediated ablation in spine interventional procedures (Fig. 6.1).

Mechanism of Action

- Plasma-mediated ablation belongs to standard electrosurgical techniques, and is already widely used in ear, nose, and throat surgery for tonsillectomy and adenoidectomy, and sports medicine for arthroplasty and meniscectomy. However, the technology has been recently introduced in the field of percutaneous tissue ablative techniques, mainly for interventional spine procedures. Its main advantage is that it achieves volumetric removal of target tissue at cooler temperatures than other ablative techniques like radiofrequency and microwave ablation.

K. Katsanos, M.Sc., M.D., Ph.D., EBIR
Department of Interventional Radiology, Patras University Hospital (PGNP),
Panepistimiou Street, Rion, Patras 26504, Greece
e-mail: katsanos@med.upatras.gr

T. Clark, T. Sabharwal (eds.), *Interventional Radiology Techniques in Ablation*,
Techniques in Interventional Radiology,
DOI 10.1007/978-0-85729-094-6_6, © Springer-Verlag London 2013

Fig. 6.1 Plasma-radiofrequency ablation electrode. Note the *yellow glow* emitted by the energized plasma field formed at the tip of the device operating within a saline environment (Courtesy of ArthroCare, US, by permission)

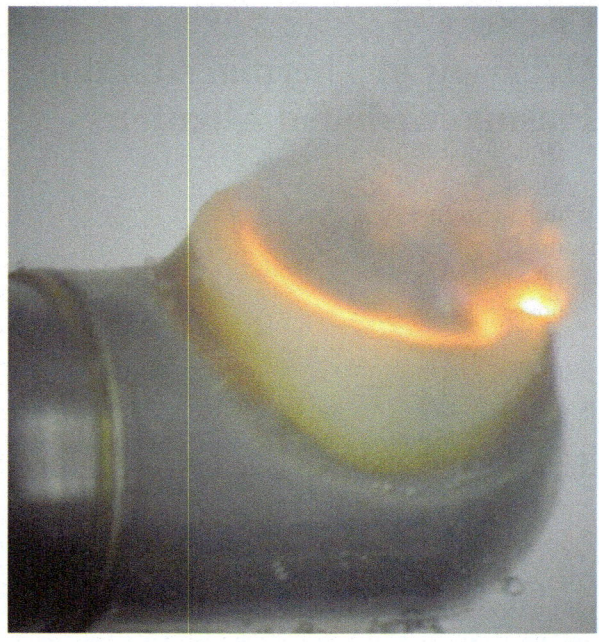

- In principle, delivery of voltage-mediated bipolar radiofrequency energy from the source electrode excites the ions of surrounding electrolytic solutions and produces a precisely focused plasma ion field delivered at the tip of the active electrode. The ionization process consumes most of the generated heat, and no electrical current passes directly through the target tissue. In physics and chemistry, plasma is a state of matter similar to gas in which a certain portion of the particles is ionized.

- Plasma has properties quite unlike those of solids, liquids, or gases and is therefore considered a distinct state of matter, in which many electrons are free and unbound and move independently. According to basic physics, "plasma" is defined as "a collection of charged particles containing about equal numbers of positive ions and electrons and exhibiting some properties of a gas but differing from a gas in being a good conductor of electricity and in being affected by a magnetic field" (Merriam-Webster Online Dictionary 2009).

- Coblation technology harnesses this physics phenomenon by applying local bipolar radiofrequency energy. Basically, coblation generates an electric field between two small electrodes; i.e. electrical current flows through an electrically conductive solution to excite electrolytes and molecules creating high-density energy field or ion plasma. The electrical current flows between an active electrode located on the tip of a radiofrequency device and a return electrode located more proximally on the same device (bipolar radiofrequency electrode). Presence of an electrolytic solution, such as normal saline, is necessary for operation of the electrical circuit, formation of a local gas layer (by radiofrequency overheating), and subsequent ionization (i.e. loss of electrons) of available gaseous microparticles.

- Within saline-type environments, the electrical excitation can range from low-voltage, non-plasma-forming tissue-heating conditions (causing tissue coagulation to achieve hemostasis, for example) to higher-voltage plasma-forming conditions that can cut or excise tissue rapidly with minimal collateral tissue damage. Radiofrequency excitation frequencies employed for Coblation devices commonly range from 100 to 500 kHz.

- Nonplasma settings: At lower voltages, typically below about 65–125 V, the saline solution is merely activated by joule dissipation of the electrolyte ions moving in the solution in response to the imposed electric fields. This heated fluid can interact with nearby tissue. If the tissue is electrically conductive enough (usually through the presence of naturally occurring electrolytes such as sodium, potassium, and chloride), it can also be heated directly by the electrical currents. Blood vessels within the tissue may also be coagulated, thereby stopping their bleeding during the procedure.

- Plasma settings: With plasma ablation settings, a higher voltage (150–350 V) is introduced across the bipolar electrodes. This electrical field interacts with underlying fluid, such as saline, to excite electrolytes and molecules in the fluid and create a high-density energy ion plasma field. The formation of a gas layer is an important first process leading to the plasma-forming conditions. Gas formation at the tip of the electrodes is the result of an electrochemical process at the surface of the electrodes. When the local joule heating of the saline induced by the electric field and current density near the energized electrodes exceeds the heat of vaporization of the fluid (e.g. water) and the rate at which the heat dissipates due to thermal conduction, localized vaporization can develop. As a very thin vapor layer forms (on the order of 100 µm) and high impedance of the vapor layer when compared with the saline occurs, the electric field across this area, which is localized in thin regions around the electrode(s), increases dramatically (300 V across 100 µm is 30,000 V/cm), ionizing and fragmenting the water molecules in the vapor layer and forming the plasma field.

- Once in plasma mode, thermal power is reduced while the plasma ablative effectiveness intensifies due to increased chemical activity driven by the higher electron energy. This increased electron energy is a result of electron acceleration (movement) induced by the higher electric field in the plasma. The ionized plasma field glows yellow in the presence of excited sodium (Na) atoms from the NaCl-based saline solution used to generate the plasma and has a depth of approximately 100–200 µm (as thick as a sheet of paper). Generally, the glow color depends on the ions of the electrolytic medium. For example, the tip will have a pinkish-blue glow, which is characteristic of excited potassium (K) atoms, in the presence of a potassium chloride (KCl) based medium.

- The plasma field acts like a condensator breaking down the intramolecular connections in biological tissues producing tissue cavitation and effective tumor debulking and decompression. Plasma-mediated disintegration of tissue produces elementary molecules that are evacuated through the puncture needle mainly in the form of low molecular weight gases, i.e. nitrogen, carbon dioxide, etc.

- Plasma-mediated ablation produces only a slight increase in temperature around the electrode, which does not exceed 80°C. It therefore functions at much cooler temperatures (typically 40–70°C vs. 400–600°C for ordinary electrocautery ablation). This is why it is otherwise known as cool ablation or coblation. Tissue ablation by the ionized plasma field at relatively low temperatures avoids excessive heat damage and preserves the integrity of surrounding healthy tissues. However, serious nerve injury may occur from direct contact of the tip of the activated plasma electrode with a nerve root or the spinal cord.

- Existing coblation technology combines two modes of action: first tissue ablation via molecular dissociation and second tissue coagulation via localized resistive heating. Tissue cavitation is performed during forward advancement of the electrode and tissue coagulation during electrode retraction. Therefore, plasma-mediated coblation involves continuous back-and-forth movements in conjunction with axial rotational steering of an S-shaped plasma electrode in order to create multiple channels within the lesion of interest. The higher the number of channels, the greater the volume of tissue destruction and cavitation.

Indications for Use

- Percutaneous discectomy/nucleoplasty in case of chronic discogenic back pain and failure of conservative therapy. Indications include symptomatic disk protrusions and contained disk hernias of the cervical and lumbar spine producing axial and/or radicular pain. Plasma-RF cavitation of the disk nucleus pulposus aims in volumetric tissue reduction of the disk hernia and effective decompression of the afflicted nerve roots. Treatment of extruded disk fragments and disk sequestrations is contra-indicated at the moment.
- Tumor decompression in case of malignant metastatic disease of the spine and pelvis. Goal of therapy is palliative local debulking of neoplastic tissue to avert compression of sensitive neurological structures, mainly the spinal cord. Best candidates for plasma-mediated ablation are nonsurgical patients suffering from painful spinal tumors with intracanalar bulge or rupture of the vertebral posterior wall with increased risk of tumor retropulsion during standard vertebroplasty. The technique aims pain management with a combination of tumor reduction, tissue decompression, and bone consolidation.
- Similar to kyphoplasty, plasma cavitation of the vertebral bodies or other spinal lesions has been also proposed before vertebroplasty in order to reduce the associated risk of cement leakage during vertebral consolidation with cementoplasty.

Image Guidance and Lesion Access

- Place the patient in the prone position for routine spinal interventional procedures. Insert soft pillows below the lower abdomen and below the lower legs to comfortably straighten the spine.
- Coblation treatment is usually well tolerated with routine conscious sedation or neuroleptanalgesia. General anesthesia is seldom necessary.

- Needle insertion is typically performed under routine cross-sectional or fluoroscopic guidance. Use routine local anesthesia with 1% lidocaine, combination of opiate (fentanyl) and midazolam, and/or propofol anesthesia titrated to avoid respiratory failure.
- High-quality single-plane or biplane fluoroscopy with or without adjunctive CT imaging is the preferred mode of guidance for spinal procedures.
- Computed tomography (CT) has high spatial resolution, which is of crucial importance for the targeting of spinal and pelvic lesions located near sensitive neuroaxial structures. Thin-section CT to allow for multiplanar reformatting and/ or biplane high-quality fluoroscopy is recommended in order to achieve optimal lesion targeting and minimize complications.
- Choose the shortest and safest needle path after careful review of the preprocedure CT scan. Route of access may be standard transpedicular, intercostovertebral, parapedicular, paravertebral, or other custom site access.
- Angling of the computed tomography scanner gantry may aid accessibility if traditional orthogonal axial views fail to show a safe route of access.
- CT fluoroscopy is an emerging adjunctive tool for high-precision real-time guided targeting of lesions that are difficult to access. Scanning parameters must be carefully adjusted to minimize radiation exposure.

Treatment Application

- Use a dedicated bipolar electrode capable of producing an ion plasma field inserted into the tumor or disk with a co-axial technique through a larger cannula, typically a bone trocar.
- There are 17–19G electrodes dedicated for percutaneous nucleoplasty and 8–11G electrodes dedicated for percutaneous spinal tumor decompression.
- A side-arm catheter is connected to the electrode to allow for slow injection of an electrolytic solution, usually normal saline, for creation of the energized ion plasma field.
- Under fluoroscopy, 180° axial rotation and back-and-forth motion of a plasma-RF electrode with a bent tip achieves digging of multiple channels inside the disk or tumor with effective tissue decompression. Avoid ablating near the vertebral bone endplates and near the spinal canal or exiting nerve roots.
- Goal of treatment is to vaporize and cavitate the nucleus pulposus in case of symptomatic disk hernias and most of the central tumor core in case of malignancy in order to achieve volumetric target tissue reduction.
- The procedure can be followed by other complimentary vertebral augmentation procedures such as vertebroplasty or kyphoplasty for cement bone consolidation.
- Safety of plasma-RF ablative procedures may be enhanced with the use of appropriate thermo-sensors and insulation techniques. Thermo-sensors can be inserted near sensitive neurovascular or visceral structures for temperature monitoring.

- Carbon dioxide insufflation, in particular, can be very useful for displacement of vital hollow organs and protection of adjacent nerve structures because of its high insulation coefficient and absent risk of embolism.
- Immediately abort the ablative process if the patient complains of sudden onset of pain. Confirm proper placement of the active electrode inside the target lesion under fluoroscopy. NEVER activate the electrode without proper fluoroscopic control.

Treatment Outcomes

- Plasma-RF ablation procedures are usually performed on an outpatient basis under local anesthesia and sedation with minimal major safety concerns.
- In case of percutaneous disc nucleoplasty, complete resolution or significant improvement in symptoms has been reported in 50–70% of the cases for at 1 year.
- In case of percutaneous tumor decompression of painful spine malignancies, significant pain relief has been reported in >90% of the cases in low-volume series.
- Long-term and comparative data about plasma-RF ablation are missing.

Complications

- Inadvertent damage of adjacent sensitive organs (spinal cord, nerve roots, ureter, bladder, or bowel)
- Internal hemorrhage, subdural/epidural hematoma

Key Points
- The plasma field is a distinct state of matter characterized by a highly ionized gas, consisting of free electrons, ions, and excited radicals.
- Energized plasma ion particles are sufficiently (re)active to disintegrate organic molecular bonds of biological tissue into elementary molecules. Thus, the target tissue is effectively dissolved or cavitated at relatively low temperatures with minimal damage to surrounding healthy tissues.
- Plasma-RF ablative technology is more precise in dissolving tissue and functions at cooler temperatures than other radiofrequency-based technologies, generating tissue temperatures of 40–70°C versus other technologies such as electrocautery that produce tissue temperatures of 400–600°C.
- Within the context of spine interventional procedures, indications for volumetric tissue reduction by plasma-RF ablation include percutaneous nucleoplasty in case of symptomatic disk hernias of the cervical and lumbar spine, and tumor decompression in case of painful nonsurgical malignancies of the spine and pelvis.

- Low-temperature plasma electrocautery minimizes bleeding
- Local infection and/or abscess or fistula formation

Suggested Reading

Birnbaum K. Percutaneous cervical disc decompression. Surg Radiol Anat. 2009;31(5):379–87.

Carrafiello G, Laganà D, Pellegrino C, Fontana F, Mangini M, Nicotera P, Petullà M, Bracchi E, Genovese E, Cuffari S, Fugazzola C. Percutaneous imaging-guided ablation therapies in the treatment of symptomatic bone metastases: preliminary experience. Radiol Med. 2009;114(4):608–25.

Georgy BA, Wong W. Plasma-mediated radiofrequency ablation assisted percutaneous cement injection for treating advanced malignant vertebral compression fractures. AJNR Am J Neuroradiol. 2007;28:700–5.

Gerszten PC, Monaco 3rd EA. Complete percutaneous treatment of vertebral body tumors causing spinal canal compromise using a transpedicular cavitation, cement augmentation, and radiosurgical technique. Neurosurg Focus. 2009;27(6):E9.

Gerszten PC, Smuck M, Rathmell JP, Simopoulos TT, Bhagia SM, Mocek CK, Crabtree T, Bloch DA, SPINE Study Group. Plasma disc decompression compared with fluoroscopy-guided transforaminal epidural steroid injections for symptomatic contained lumbar disc herniation: a prospective, randomized, controlled trial. J Neurosurg Spine. 2010;12(4):357–71.

Stalder KR, McMillen DF, Woloszko J. Electrosurgical plasmas. J Phys D Appl Phys. 2005;38: 1728–38.

Part II
Clinical Applications

Chapter 7
Radiofrequency Ablation of Thyroid and Parathyroid Nodules

Jung Hwan Baek

Clinical Features

- Thyroid nodules are very common in adults, found in 4–8% by palpation, in 10–41% by ultrasonography (US), and in 50% by pathologic examination at autopsy.
- Most thyroid nodules are benign. Whereas the majority of nodules do not require treatment, some may need it, for various reasons including pressure symptoms and cosmetic problems.
- Patients with autonomously functioning thyroid nodules (AFTNs) may have subclinical hyperthyroidism, with approximately 4% per year progressing to obvious hyperthyroidism or thyrotoxicosis. These conditions may have detrimental effects on the skeletal (osteoporosis) and cardiovascular (atrial fibrillation) systems. Large AFTNs may result in clinical problems similar to those of benign cold nodules, such as cosmetic problems and pressure symptoms.
- Repeat surgery in the central or lateral compartments of the neck may be difficult in patients with recurrent thyroid cancer because previous neck dissection may be associated with high rates of morbidity.
- Hyperparathyroidism is a major problem in patients with parathyroid nodules. Secondary hyperparathyroidism is caused by chronic dialysis in patients with chronic renal failure. Long-standing hyperparathyroidism causes cardiovascular disease, hypertension, renal stones, osteoporosis, and bone pain. Large parathyroid nodules may cause neck discomfort and cosmetic problems.

J.H. Baek, M.D.
Department of Radiology and Research Institute of Radiology,
University of Ulsan College of Medicine, Asan Medical Center,
86 Asanbyeongwon-Gil, Songpa-gu, Seoul 138-736, Korea
e-mail: radbaek@naver.com, www.gap.kr

T. Clark, T. Sabharwal (eds.), *Interventional Radiology Techniques in Ablation*,   53
Techniques in Interventional Radiology,
DOI 10.1007/978-0-85729-094-6_7, © Springer-Verlag London 2013

Diagnostic Evaluation

Clinical

- Have patients rate their symptoms using a 10-cm visual analog scale [1–4].
- Have physicians sort patients into those with four categories of cosmetic problems [1–4]:
  1. No palpable mass
  2. No cosmetic problem but palpable mass
  3. Cosmetic problem on swallowing only
  4. Readily detected cosmetic problem
- Assess clinical symptoms related to thyroid function abnormality (e.g., tachycardia, atrial fibrillation, fatigue, asthenia, emotional lability, and dyspnea).
- Evaluate clinical symptoms related to hyperparathyroidism (e.g., easy fatigue, bone pain, depression, acid reflux, high blood pressure, renal stones, thinning hair, palpitations, and osteoporosis).

Laboratory

The following parameters should be assessed before radiofrequency (RF) ablation is considered:
- CBC
- Blood coagulation test
- Thyrotropin (TSH), thyroid hormone, and thyroid autoantibody levels
- Calcitonin level
- Thyroglobulin level in patients with recurrent thyroid cancer after total thyroidectomy
- Parathyroid hormone, calcium, and phosphate levels, to diagnose hyperparathyroidism

Imaging

- Preprocedural US examination should be performed to evaluate thyroid nodules and to plan RF ablation:

  - Size – calculated by measuring three orthogonal diameters of each nodule
  - Volume – calculated using the equation: $V = \pi abc/6$ (V volume, a the largest diameter, b and c the other two perpendicular diameters)
  - Characteristics of the nodules (shape, margin, internal content, echogenicity, and calcifications)

- Composition – classified as solid (having a solid portion >90%), predominantly solid (having a solid portion >50%), predominantly cystic (having a cystic portion >50%), or cystic (having a cystic portion >90%)
- Vascularity – classified as vascular status in <25%, 25–50%, 50–75%, or >75% of the nodule
- Presence of abnormal lymph nodes in the neck
- Relationship between the target nodule (or recurrent cancer) and critical neck structures (vessels, trachea, recurrent laryngeal nerve, esophagus, vagus nerve, phrenic nerve, and sympathetic chain)

- [^{99m}Tc] pertechnetate scintigraphy may be helpful in differentiating cold nodules from AFTNs in some patients with elevated serum TSH.
- A neck CT scan may be useful to evaluate the intrathoracic extent of benign thyroid nodules and the degree of recurrent thyroid cancer.
- A parathyroid scan and US examination are essential to localize targeted parathyroid nodules. CT or an MRI scan may also be required to evaluate ectopic mediastinal parathyroid nodules.

Indications

- Benign nodules diagnosed by fine-needle aspiration cytology (FNAC) at two separate times and showing no malignant US features [5, 6].

    - Subjective symptoms (pain, discomfort, swallowing difficulty, and pressure symptoms)
    - Cosmetic problems
    - AFTN

- Recurrent thyroid cancer: patients who are poor candidates for surgery or who refuse to undergo surgery.
- Parathyroid adenoma: patients who are poor candidates for surgery or who refuse to undergo surgery.

Contraindications

Absolute

- There are no absolute contraindications.
- However, RF ablation is not recommended for patients with thyroid cancer (primary or recurrent) who are good candidates for surgery.

Relative Contraindications

- Bleeding tendency
- Contralateral vocal cord palsy
- Follicular neoplasm

Patient Preparation

- Patients are allowed to drink clear fluids up to the time of the procedure, but should have no solid food for at least 6 h before a procedure.
- Patients should be given an information leaflet, so that they can learn about the technique, the surgical aims, and potential complications.
- Patients should be aware that the therapeutic response to RF ablation is gradual.
- A venous line should be established in the antecubital vein of the arm, which is the preferred route of drug delivery (e.g., for control of pain or hypertension).
- Thermal ablation has been classified as a procedure carrying a high risk of bleeding [7]. Patients taking aspirin or antiplatelet drugs should be told to discontinue such medication 7–10 days before RF ablation, and patients taking warfarin should be told to cease taking the drug 3–5 days before ablation. However, physicians should weigh the benefits of RF ablation against potential complications related to interruption of aspirin, warfarin, or antiplatelet drugs, and, if needed, should consider hospitalization or use of parenteral anticoagulation therapy [7].

Relevant Anatomy

Normal Anatomy

- The thyroid gland lies anterior and lateral to the trachea in the visceral space of infrahyoid neck.
- The common carotid artery and the internal jugular vein are located posterolaterally to the thyroid gland.
- The infrahyoid strap muscles are located anteriorly to the thyroid gland.
- The sternocleidomastoid muscles are located anterolaterally to the thyroid gland.
- The parathyroid glands, usually four in number, lie close to the deep surface of the thyroid gland. Normal parathyroid glands are ovoid in shape and approximately 4–6 mm in length, with the inferior glands being larger than the superior glands. The location of the superior parathyroid glands, relative to the thyroid gland, is more constant than is that of the inferior parathyroid glands.
- The superior thyroidal artery runs superficially on the anterior border of the thyroid gland. This artery is closely associated with and anterolateral to the external branch of the superior laryngeal nerve.

- The interior thyroidal artery enters the tracheo-esophageal groove in a plane posterior to the carotid space and branches thereof penetrate the posterior aspect of the lateral thyroid lobe.
- Many delicate structures are located around the thyroid gland and in the neck.

  - The recurrent laryngeal nerve is located on the right posteromedial aspect of the trachea and the left tracheo-esophageal groove.
  - The esophagus is usually located on the left posteromedial aspect of the trachea.
  - Trachea.
  - The common carotid artery and internal jugular vein are located in the posterolateral aspect of the thyroid gland.
  - The vagus nerve, located posterolateral to the common carotid artery and posteromedial to the internal jugular vein, is easily detected on US using a linear probe.
  - The anterior jugular vein begins near the hyoid bone at the confluence of several superficial veins arising from the submaxillary region. The vein descends along the anterior border of the sternocleidomastoid muscle and passes beneath that muscle to open into the external jugular vein in the lower part of the neck. This vein is located along the approach route (in front of the isthmus) of the electrode.
  - The brachial plexus runs from the spine and is formed by the ventral rami of the lower four cervical and first thoracic nerve roots (C5-T1). The roots of the brachial plexus are posterior to the thyroid gland. Therefore, a posteriorly bulging thyroid mass may be very close to the brachial plexus.
  - The phrenic nerve descends obliquely with the internal jugular vein across the anterior scalene muscle. On the left, the phrenic nerve crosses anterior to the first part of the subclavian artery. On the right, the phrenic nerve lies on the anterior scalene muscle and crosses anterior to the second part of the subclavian artery. On both sides, the phrenic nerve runs posterior to the subclavian vein and anterior to the internal thoracic artery as the nerve enters the thorax.
  - The cervical sympathetic trunk, which is ventral to the transverse process of the cervical vertebra and close to the carotid artery, is located in the carotid sheath or in the connective tissue between the sheath and the longus colli/capitis muscle.

Aberrant Anatomy

- Anterior and medial variations of the vagus nerve may be located very close or attached to the thyroid gland and/or the targeted thyroid nodule [8–10].
- Right-sided esophagus: Although the esophagus is usually located on the left, it can be located on the right.
- An aberrant recurrent laryngeal nerve is usually detected on the right side, associated with an aberrant right subclavian artery. If the latter is suspected, the physician should remember that the aberrant recurrent laryngeal nerve can also be located on the right.

- The far-lateral portion of the normal thyroid gland may extend to the area between the common carotid artery and the internal jugular vein. Thyroid nodules arising from this portion may be very close to the vagus nerve.
- Inferior parathyroid glands are more commonly in aberrant locations than are superior parathyroid glands. The aberrant locations of the former include the mediastinum, the carotid artery bifurcation, within the carotid sheath, and the intrathyroid, retroesophageal, and retropharyngeal areas.

Equipment

Generator

- An RF generator supplies RF power to the tissue through an electrode.

Electrode

- Internally cooled electrode [1–4, 11–13].
  - Conventional straight type (17-gauge; 15 cm in length; 1-cm active tip).
  - Modified straight type (18-gauge; 7 cm in length; 0.5-, 0.7-, 1-, or 1.5-cm sized active tips). Modified electrodes are short (7 cm), to permit easy control, and thin (18-gauge), to minimize injury to the normal thyroid gland [2]. Small-sized (0.5- and 0.7-cm) active tips have been used to treat small recurrent thyroid cancers [14].
- Multitined expandable electrodes (14-gauge; 10 cm in length; bearing 4–9 hooks expandable to 3.5–4 cm) have been used in Italy [15, 16].

Grounding Pads

- Grounding pads act to disperse electricity in an RF circuit.

Pump

- A peristaltic pump is used to perfuse cool water through the perfusion port of the electrode, preventing vaporization and carbonization.

Preprocedure Medications

- Premedication is generally not required.
- For patients on warfarin, see the section on "patient preparation."

Procedure

Patient

- Patients are placed in the supine position with mild neck extension.
- Two grounding pads are attached firmly to both thighs.
- Lidocaine (2%, w/v) is used for local anesthesia of the puncture site and around the thyroid gland and/or thyroid nodule.
- The skin is not incised, thus preventing unnecessary scar formation.

Planning an Access Route

- Careful observation of the vessels along the approach route is required to prevent the electrode from causing serious hemorrhage.
- Three approach methods have been developed:
- *Trans-isthmic approach method* [1, 3, 4, 12, 17]:

  - The electrode approach is made from the medial (isthmus) to the lateral (nodule) aspect along the transverse axis of the targeted nodule (Fig. 7.1).
  - The entire length of the electrode and the tip can be easily visualized on the transverse US view (Fig. 7.2a). This allows visualization of the relationship

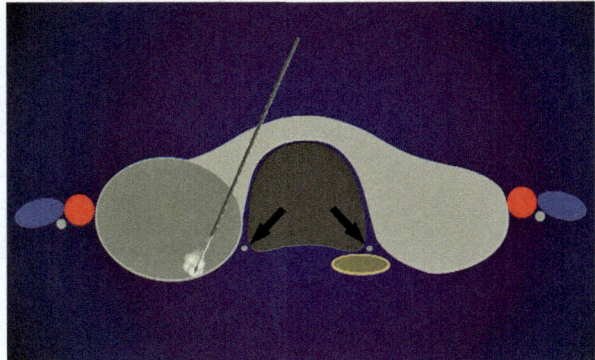

Fig. 7.1 Diagram of the trans-isthmic approach method. The electrode approaches from the medial (the isthmus) region in the direction of the lateral aspect (the nodule). The electrode passes through an amount of normal thyroid parenchyma (in the isthmus) sufficient to steady the needle. The thyroid nodule is very close to the recurrent laryngeal nerve (*arrows*), trachea, and vessels

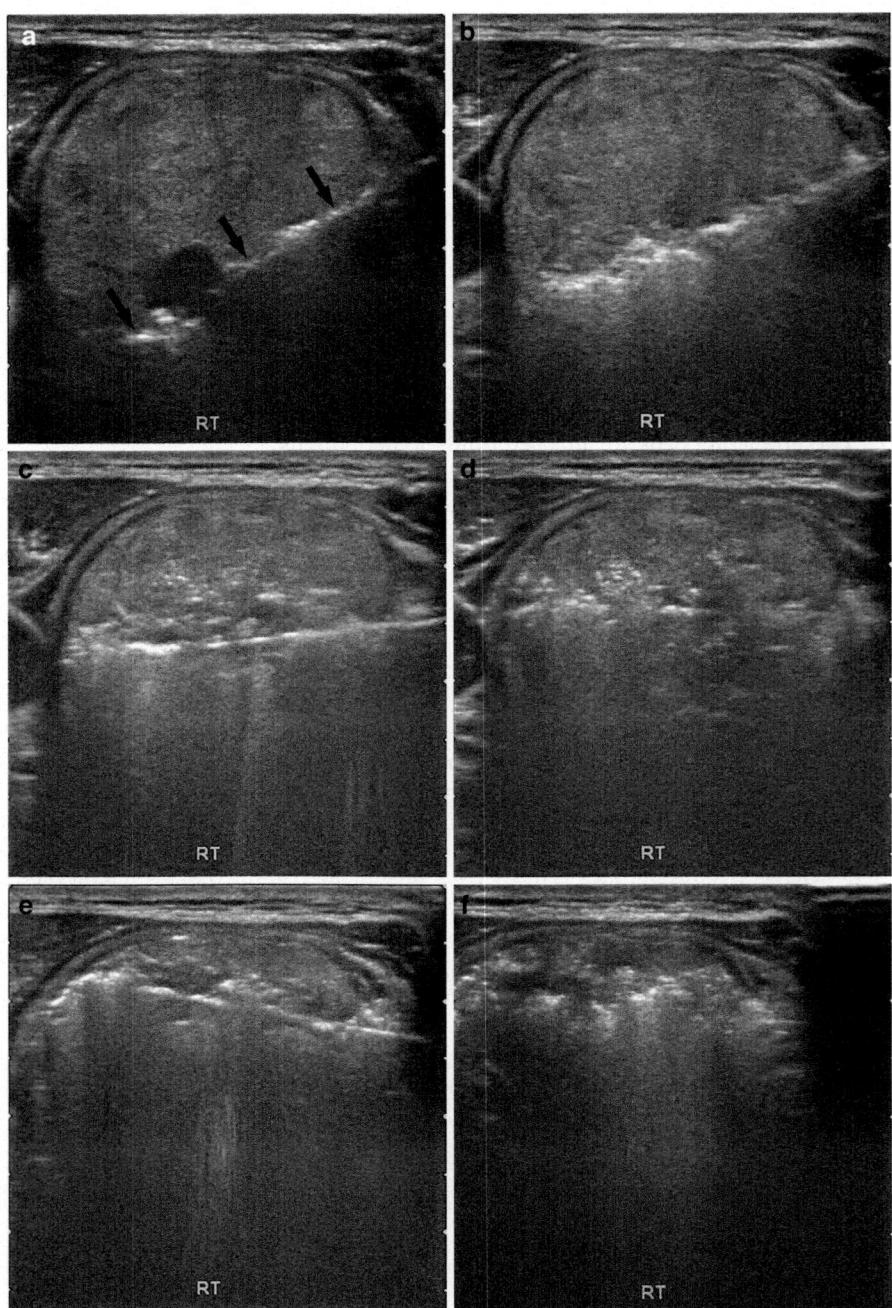

Fig. 7.2 Sequential ultrasonographic images of the moving shot technique. (**a**) On a transverse ultrasonographic view, and using the trans-isthmic approach, the entire length of the electrode and the tip thereof can be easily visualized (*arrows*). Initially, the tip is positioned in the deepest, most remote portion of the tumor, enabling the tip to be easily monitored without disturbances caused by microbubbles. (**b**–**e**) When a transient echogenic area appears in the targeted ablating unit, the electrode is continuously moved backward and in the superficial direction to treat other ablation units. (**f**) When all conceptual ablation units of the targeted nodule have changed to transient hyperechoic zones, RF ablation is terminated

among the electrode tip, the thyroid nodule, the trachea, and the great vessels, and may also be used to locate the recurrent laryngeal nerve. Clear visualization of the relationship between the electrode tip and these structures may prevent complications.

- Passing the electrode through a sufficient amount of thyroid parenchyma (in the isthmus) may prevent the position of the electrode tip from moving during swallowing or talking, and may also prevent leakage of hot ablated fluid outside the thyroid gland.

- *Cranio-caudal (longitudinal) approach method* [15, 16]:

    - The electrode approach is made from the superior to the inferior aspect of a targeted nodule along the long axis of the nodule. It is difficult to determine the relationship between the electrode tip and delicate structures in the neck. Frequently, movement of the electrode is limited by the mandible or clavicle.

- *Lateral approach method*:

    - If many enlarged vessels are present in the isthmus, the lateral approach method may prevent serious hemorrhage.

Ablation Technique: Moving Shot Approach

- The moving shot technique for thyroid RF ablation was designed to avoid thermal injury to surrounding structures [1–4, 11, 12] (Fig. 7.2).
- The basic ablation technique for liver tumors requires that the electrode be fixed during ablation. The ablation technique for thyroid nodules should differ from that used to treat the liver tumors.
- The thyroid gland is smaller than the liver, and thyroid nodules are usually ellipsoid in shape rather than round (liver tumors). Therefore, prolonged fixation of the electrode during ablation of thyroid nodules may damage surrounding delicate structures.
- Conceptual ablating units: The thyroid nodule is divided into several conceptual ablating units of various sizes.

    - These conceptual ablating units are smaller at the periphery of the nodule or in areas adjacent to the delicate structures of the neck.
    - The conceptual ablating units are larger in the central safer portion of the nodule.
    - RF ablation should be performed unit-by-unit by moving the electrode (Fig. 7.2).

- The moving shot technique should be used, together with an internally cooled electrode, because this type of electrode minimizes charring and is easy to move continuously.

- Such electrodes have 1- and 1.5-cm active tips for treatment of benign thyroid nodules and 0.5-, 0.7-, and 1-cm tips for use in treatment of recurrent thyroid cancers.
- Ablation is commenced with 10 W (0.5-cm active tip), 20 W (0.7-cm active tip), 30 W (1-cm active tip), or 50 W (1.5-cm active tip) of RF power under the impedance control mode.
- If a transient hyperechoic zone at the electrode tip does not appear within 5–10 s, RF power is increased in 10 W increments up to 100–110 W. During ablation, RF power level is dictated principally by the internal structure of the targeted nodule.
- Initially, the electrode tip is positioned in the deepest, most remote portion of the nodule, to enable easy monitoring of the electrode tip without disturbances caused by microbubbles. When a transient echogenic area appears in the targeted ablating unit, the electrode is continuously moved backward and in the superficial direction, to enter untreated ablating units (Fig. 7.2).
- In instances of predominantly cystic thyroid nodules, cystic fluid should be aspirated prior to ablation of the solid portion.
- If a patient experiences intolerable pain during RF ablation, the power should be reduced or turned off for several seconds. Pain or discomfort usually dissipates rapidly and the procedure may then be continued.
- Voice change should be checked intermittently during the procedure.
- Total ablation time usually ranges from 10 to 20 min for a 3–4-cm-diameter nodule, but ablation time depends on the experience of the operator.

Endpoint of the Procedure

- The endpoint of the procedure is when all conceptual ablating units of the targeted nodule, whether benign or malignant, have changed to transient hyperechoic zones (Fig. 7.2f).
- A small portion of a nodule may remain undertreated in some patients for the following reasons:

  - An area of a thyroid nodule may lie very close to critical structures such as the recurrent laryngeal nerve, trachea, or esophagus.
  - A nodule may be too large for complete ablation in one session.
  - Intrathoracic extension of a thyroid nodule: The far-inferior portion of the nodule may not be visible by US.

Immediate Postprocedure Care

- Operators should check for possible complications, such as bleeding at the puncture site or voice problems.
- The puncture site should be compressed mildly for 10–20 min to prevent hemorrhage.

- Thyroid RF ablation is basically an outpatient procedure. After observing patients in the hospital for 1 h, they can be discharged.
- Laboratory tests before discharge from the hospital:

  - Patients with benign thyroid nodules: TSH and thyroid hormone levels.
  - Patients with parathyroid nodules: Parathyroid hormone, calcium, and phosphate levels.

Follow-up and Postprocedure Medications

- The physician should explore the following aspects at follow-up visits:

  - Any complications or complaints.
  - Volume and ablation status of the nodule.
  - Status of clinical problems: cosmetic and symptomatic issues.
  - Blood examination: A repeat blood examination is required if the serum concentration of thyroid hormone was abnormal immediately after RF ablation. Repeat blood examinations are usually required for patients with AFTN and recurrent cancer.

- Imaging tools: US is the primary examination tool, with CT and [99mTc] pertechnetate scintigraphy serving in ancillary roles.
- Follow-up intervals: Patients are usually followed-up at 1, 3, 6, and 12 months after the procedure, and every 6–12 months during the second year after ablation.
- US findings of successful ablation [12] (Fig. 7.3):

  - Loss of intranodular vascular signal in Doppler US examination.
  - Decreased nodule volume.
  - Decreased echogenicity of the ablated nodule (which can now look like a malignancy).

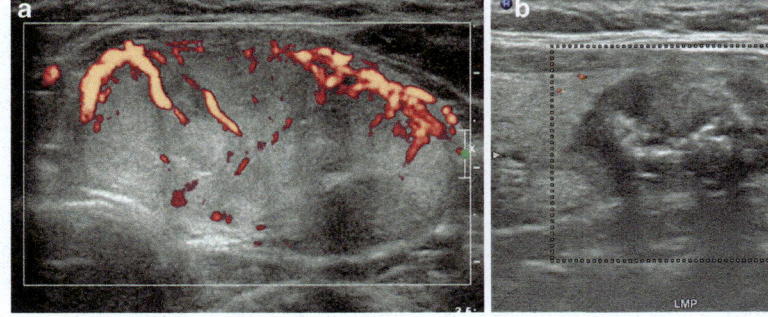

Fig. 7.3 Ultrasound findings of successful ablation. (**a**) Before ablation, a large isoechoic left thyroid nodule with internal vascularity is visible. (**b**) Sixteen months after RF ablation, the successfully ablated nodule shows loss of intranodular vascular signals, marked nodule volume reduction, and decreased echogenicity. Sometimes, development of intranodular calcifications can be detected

- Changes in size, echogenicity, and intranodular vascularity of the nodule should be evaluated on follow-up US examinations.
- Volume reduction (VR) is calculated using the following equation:

$$VR\,(\%) = \left[\text{initial volume (ml)} - \text{final volume (ml)}\right] \times 100\,/\,\text{initial volume}$$

- Patients with intrathoracic extension of the thyroid nodule or recurrent cancer may require CT examination for comparison with CT data obtained before the procedure.
- Clinical changes in pressure symptoms and cosmetic problem scores should be evaluated serially on follow-up visits.
- On the day after ablation, neck bulging may be aggravated and the volume of the ablated nodule may increase. These findings are caused by edema and swelling of the ablated nodule and surrounding soft tissue. Volume reduction usually commences 3–7 days after ablation, with the greatest reduction in volume observed at the 1-month follow-up, followed by a subsequent further gradual reduction.
- If serum concentrations of TSH and thyroid hormones remain abnormal after RF ablation, these materials should be re-assayed at the 1-month follow-up. Regular measurement of TSH and thyroid hormone levels are essential to determine the amount of antithyroid drug to administer after RF ablation of AFTN.
- Follow-up US examination is usually not required when the treated nodule shows sufficient volume reduction without evidence of a remaining untreated portion.
- [99mTc] pertechnetate scintigraphy, blood, and US examinations are essential to evaluate the ablation status of AFTN. US examination and laboratory tests for TSH and thyroid hormone should be performed 1, 3, 6, and 12 months after RF ablation. Measurements of thyroid autoantibodies and [99mTc] pertechnetate scintigraphy should be performed 6 months after RF ablation [2].
- For patients with recurrent thyroid cancer, US examinations should be performed at 1, 3, 6, and 12 months, and thyroglobulin concentration should be measured at 6 months, after RF ablation. CT scans at 1 month are recommended to evaluate the status of ablated thyroid cancers. Completely ablated cancers show no enhancing portion on follow-up CT scans. Such scans may also detect newly developed recurrent cancers. In some instances, the degree of enhancement on CT is more useful than is US in evaluating the ablation status of recurrent cancers.
- Patients who undergo RF ablation of parathyroid nodules should undergo US examination, parathyroid scanning, and blood testing at follow-up visits.
- Additional RF ablation [1, 2, 12]:

  - If a nodule is too large to be ablated completely in a single session, a second RF ablation may be scheduled 1–2 months later, because reduction in nodule volume is rapid during the first month after RF ablation.

- If hyperfunctioning thyroid or parathyroid nodules are not corrected, additional ablation is required as soon as possible.
- If follow-up US shows that a portion of the nodule is viable (i.e., the echogenicity is equal to that of the index nodule and intranodular vascularity is evident), and patients complain of incompletely resolved clinical problems, additional RF ablation is indicated.
- If follow-up US results suggest regrowth of an untreated peripheral portion of the nodule, an additional RF ablation should be scheduled. The tendency to regrow is relatively high for treated nodules with abundant peripheral vascularity.

- Usually, postprocedure medication is not required. Patients who complain of pain or discomfort may benefit from treatment with oral analgesics (acetaminophen).

Results

The results of RF ablation of benign nodules are evaluated by changes in volume and clinical problems (pressure symptoms and cosmetic issues), as well as by changes in serum concentration of TSH and, for patients who undergo ablation of AFTNs, thyroid hormone. The results of RF ablation of recurrent thyroid cancers are evaluated by determining the extent of locoregional control of such cancers.

- A prospective randomized study comparing various treatments showed that the efficacy of RF ablation was superior to that of conservative treatment for benign, predominantly solid, nodules [1].
- Volume reduction after RF ablation ranged from 32.7% to 58.2% at 1 month and 50.7% to 84.8% at 6 months. A volume reduction greater than 50% (the therapeutic success rate) was observed for 91% of nodules, and 28% of index nodules had disappeared on follow-up US examination. After RF ablation, symptoms and cosmetic problems improved or disappeared in the majority of patients [1, 12, 13, 15, 16].
- Cosmetic and symptomatic problems are well controlled by RF ablation (Fig. 7.4).
- The efficacy of RF ablation is apparently related to nodule size, but is not affected by factors such as vascularity, amount of heat deposition, ablation time, or proportion of solid component. Ablation reduces the volume of cystic-type thyroid nodules more rapidly than those of mixed or solid-type thyroid nodules. However, 6 months after RF ablation, there was no significant difference in volume reduction among the three types of nodules [12].
- A single session of RF ablation was found to be very effective in patients with benign nonfunctioning thyroid nodules, improving both symptoms and cosmetic problems. However, large nodules may require additional treatment. Untreated peripheral portions of nodules may show regrowth on long-term follow-up; additional treatment may thus be required 1–2 years after initial RF ablation.

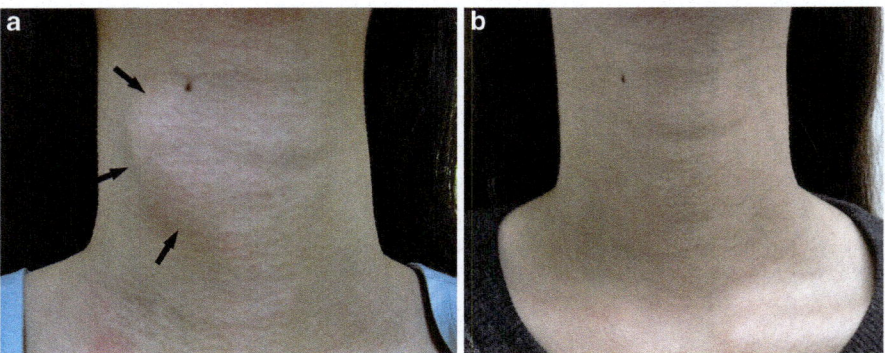

Fig. 7.4 (**a**) Photograph of a 25-year-old woman with right neck bulging caused by a large benign thyroid nodule (*arrows*). (**b**) After ablation, bulging disappeared

- RF ablation is effective in treatment of AFTN, reducing nodule volume by 70.7% at the 6-month follow-up and improving nodule-related symptoms, cosmetic problems, and abnormal thyroid function. Most patients show normalized or improved thyroid function, and the level of antithyroid drugs taken after RF ablation can be reduced [2, 16].
- Control of AFTN by RF ablation is usually more difficult than is control of cold thyroid nodules. Therefore, AFTNs may require more treatment sessions and show a greater tendency to recur [2, 15, 16]. To prevent recurrence, complete ablation is required including peripheral area of the nodules.
- RF ablation is effective in the locoregional control of recurrent cancers (88–90%), and also reduces serum thyroglobulin concentration in most patients [14, 18–20].
- To date, only two patients with hyperparathyroidism, one primary and one secondary, have been treated with RF ablation. After treatment, both patients attained normalized serum concentrations of parathyroid hormone and calcium [21, 22].

Alternative Therapies

- Surgery is a curative treatment, but has many drawbacks, such as the use of general anesthesia, voice changes, hypoparathyroidism, iatrogenic hypothyroidism, and scar formation.
- Levothyroxine medication is no longer recommended [23, 24].
- Ethanol ablation (EA):

  - EA is effective in treatment of cystic thyroid nodules, but is less effective when used to treat solid thyroid nodules.
  - For cystic thyroid nodules (cystic portion >90%), both EA and RF ablation have been found to effectively reduce nodule volume (93% vs. 92%) and to

have similar technical success rates (94.4% vs. 95.2%) in terms of improvement of both cosmetic and symptomatic problems. However, EA is superior to RF ablation with respect to the mean number of treatment sessions required (1.2 vs. 1.7) and cost. Therefore, EA may be an appropriate first-line treatment for cystic thyroid nodules [4].

- For predominantly cystic thyroid nodules (90% > cystic portion >50%), EA is less effective for nodules containing >20% of a solid portion. Therefore, RF ablation can be used for initial treatment of thyroid nodules with >20% solid component [3, 25, 26].
- For predominantly solid thyroid nodules (solid portion >50%), EA is much less effective than is RF ablation. Although additional application of EA to predominantly solid nodules may achieve efficacies similar to those obtainable with RF ablation, the complication rate increases [25].

- Percutaneous laser ablation (PLA):

  - PLA is another thermal therapeutic option for treatment of solid thyroid nodules [27–30].
  - PLA has been reported to shrink the volume of cold benign thyroid nodules by 36–82% at 6–12 month follow-up.
  - The efficacy of RF ablation appears to be slightly superior to that of PLA, and the complication rate is somewhat lower. These slight but useful benefits are attributable to use of the moving shot technique and the internal cooling system [31].
  - It should be noted, however, that several RF studies included nodules that were smaller and had a greater cystic component than had nodules treated with PLA, which were larger and more solid. Further, to date, more trial data on PLA than on RF ablation have been reported, and the former trials included more homogeneous patient groups. Thus, the accumulated evidence of efficacy is scientifically more robust for PLA than for RF ablation [31].

- High-intensity focused ultrasound (HIFU):

  - HIFU has been used to treat patients with prostate cancer, breast cancer, and uterine fibroma.
  - Animal studies applying HIFU to thyroid glands revealed destruction of particular regions of the thyroid, but skin burn was also observed [32, 33].
  - Successful HIFU ablation of a single human 0.9-cm-diameter AFTN has been reported, resulting in normalization of serum concentrations of TSH and a normal thyroid scan [34].
  - HIFU was used to treat four patients with primary hyperparathyroidism, resulting in decreased serum concentrations of parathyroid hormone in all patients, with normalization in two, and volume reductions ranging from 11% to 79%. All complications related to HIFU were transient and included mild subcutaneous edema in three patients and voice change in one [35].

Complications

- An experimental study of RF ablation on ten thyroid glands of five dogs showed various complications, including recurrent laryngeal nerve palsy in one animal, esophageal perforation in two, and esophageal wall thickening in all five [36].
- No deaths related to RF ablation have been reported.
- Pain is the most common symptom associated with the procedure. Most patients have complained of various degrees of pain at the ablated site, or pain radiating to the head, ears, shoulders, chest, back, or teeth. Pain is rapidly relieved when the RF output is reduced or turned off. Sometimes, oral painkillers are helpful in reducing pain [12].
- Esophageal perforation caused by direct thermal injury of the esophagus results in neck infection and abscess formation. This condition requires urgent surgical management.
- Voice change is one of the most serious complications of RF ablation and is caused primarily by thermal injury to the recurrent laryngeal nerve, but may also be attributable to vagus nerve injury during ablation of recurrent lateral neck lymph nodes. Frequently, an aberrant vagus nerve (in an anterior or medial location) lies very close to or in contact with the thyroid gland and targeted nodule. In this situation, voice change can be caused by injury to the vagus nerve.
- Although most patients show complete voice recovery, usually within 2–3 months, severe injury can induce permanent recurrent laryngeal nerve palsy [12, 13, 18, 19].
- Other nerve injuries: Injuries to the brachial plexus, sympathetic nerve, phrenic nerve, and spinal accessory nerve are possible, and the symptoms depend on the degree of the nerve injury:

  - Brachial plexus injury: sensory and motor disturbance of the arm and fingers.
  - Sympathetic nerve injury: Horner's syndrome.
  - Phrenic nerve injury: Elevation of the diaphragm associated with dyspnea and chest discomfort.
  - Spinal accessory nerve injury: Dysfunction of the trapezius and sternocleidomastoid muscles resulting in an asymmetric neckline, drooping shoulder, winging of the scapula, and weakness of forward head elevation.

- Thyrotoxicosis can be induced by release of thyroid hormone from thyroid follicles because of thermal and/or mechanical injury of the normal thyroid gland. However, majority of the patients do not complain of thyrotoxic symptoms. Thyrotoxicosis became normalized at the 1-month follow-up in all patients [12].
- Hypothyroidism has been reported after RF ablation of AFTN [2].
- Two types of skin burn are possible: at the electrode puncture site and at the grounding pad attachment site [13].

  - Skin burn at the puncture site is caused by direct thermal injury of overlying skin. This type of skin burn is usually first-degree, but second- and third-degree burns have been observed. Skin burns are more frequent when the thyroid nodule is large and the skin bulges.

- Skin burn at the site of grounding pad attachment site is possible, but has not yet been reported in patients undergoing thyroid RF ablation. The absence of skin burn at this site may be attributable to the relatively lower RF power (30–120 W) used for thyroid nodule ablation, compared to that employed in liver RF ablation.

- Hemorrhage is usually caused by mechanical injury to the anterior jugular vein or perithyroidal vessels. Mild compression for 5–10 min usually stops bleeding. RF ablation is usually not discontinued because of hemorrhage [12].
- Some patients have complained of nausea and vomiting after RF ablation. The cause of these symptoms is unclear. No patient to date has complained of such symptoms during ablation.
- Edema and fever are usually transient and self-limited; however, medication may be helpful to reduce such symptoms.
- Rupture of benign thyroid nodules after ablation may be caused by volume expansion resulting from delayed hemorrhage or tearing of the nodule wall. Tumor rupture should be suspected in patients who complain of sudden neck bulging or pain during follow-up periods. We recommend conservative treatment including mild compression of bulging site, without performance of invasive procedures such as needle aspiration. If symptoms progress, secondary infection may be responsible. Thus, surgical drainage or excision may be required.
- The initial symptom of tracheal thermal injury is cough. Perforation of the trachea is caused by severe thermal injury. On the left side, thermal injury to both the trachea and esophagus causes neck abscess and tracheo-esophageal fistula.
- Thermal injury to the common carotid artery and internal jugular vein is rare because of perfusion-mediated tissue cooling. However, mechanical injury caused by the electrode is possible.

How to Avoid Complications

- The operator should be aware of the exact anatomic location of adjacent critical structures, and possible associated complications.
- Use of a trans-isthmic approach and a moving shot technique may minimize possible complications [1–4, 12, 17].
- Any portion of a thyroid nodule adjacent to critical structures such as a nerve or the esophagus should be left undertreated (2–3 mm width) to prevent thermal injury.
- Swallowing of cold water during RF ablation may reduce thermal damage to the esophagus.
- Application of an ice bag to the skin can prevent skin burn.

Key Points

- RF ablation is a minimally invasive technique and a valuable alternative to surgery in treatment of benign cold thyroid nodules and AFTNs.
- RF ablation of recurrent thyroid cancers and in treatment of hyperparathyroidism may be an alternative to surgery in patients at high surgical risk.
- Use of the trans-isthmic approach and the moving shot technique are essential to ablate ellipsoid thyroid nodules completely, and to avoid thermal damage to surrounding critical structures.
- Knowledge of critical structures around the targeted lesion, and possible associated complications, is important for safe ablation.
- RF ablation of benign cold thyroid nodules shows excellent short-term results, reducing nodule volume, nodule-related symptoms, and cosmetic problems
- RF ablation of AFTNs and functioning parathyroid nodules is effective to improve function and to reduce the volume of treated nodules.
- RF ablation affords excellent locoregional control of recurrent thyroid cancers.

References

1. Baek JH, Kim YS, Lee D, Huh JY, Lee JH. Benign predominantly solid thyroid nodules: prospective study of efficacy of sonographically guided radiofrequency ablation versus control condition. AJR Am J Roentgenol. 2010;194(4):1137–42.
2. Baek JH, Moon WJ, Kim YS, Lee JH, Lee D. Radiofrequency ablation for the treatment of autonomously functioning thyroid nodules. World J Surg. 2009;33(9):1971–7.
3. Lee JH, Kim YS, Lee D, Choi H, Yoo H, Baek JH. Radiofrequency ablation (RFA) of benign thyroid nodules in patients with incompletely resolved clinical problems after ethanol ablation (EA). World J Surg. 2010;34(7):1488–93.
4. Sung JY, Kim YS, Choi H, Lee JH, Baek JH. Optimum first-line treatment technique for benign cystic thyroid nodules: ethanol ablation or radiofrequency ablation? AJR Am J Roentgenol. 2011;196(2):W210–214.
5. Moon WJ, Jung SL, Lee JH, Na DG, Baek J-H, Lee YH, et al. Benign and malignant thyroid nodules: US differentiation – multicenter retrospective study. Radiology. 2008;247(3):762–70.
6. Moon W-J, Baek JH, Jung SL, Kim DW, Kim EK, Kim JY, et al. Ultrasonography and ultrasound-based management of thyroid nodules: consensus statement and recommendations. Korean J Radiol. 2012;13(2):117–125.
7. Kwok A, Faigel DO. Management of anticoagulation before and after gastrointestinal endoscopy. Am J Gastroenterol. 2009;104(12):3085–97. quiz 98.
8. Giovagnorio F, Martinoli C. Sonography of the cervical vagus nerve: normal appearance and abnormal findings. AJR Am J Roentgenol. 2001;176(3):745–9.
9. Ha EJ, Baek JH, Lee JH, Kim JK, Shong YK. Clinical significance of vagus nerve variation in radiofrequency ablation of thyroid nodules. Eur Radiol. 2011;21(10):2151–7.
10. Park JK, Jeong SY, Lee JH, Lim GC, Chang JW. Variations in the course of the cervical vagus nerve on thyroid ultrasonography. AJNR Am J Neuroradiol. 2011;32(7):1178–1181.
11. Baek JH, Jeong HJ, Kim YS, Kwak MS, Lee D. Radiofrequency ablation for an autonomously functioning thyroid nodule. Thyroid. 2008;18(6):675–6.

12. Jeong WK, Baek JH, Rhim H, Kim YS, Kwak MS, Jeong HJ, et al. Radiofrequency ablation of benign thyroid nodules: safety and imaging follow-up in 236 patients. Eur Radiol. 2008;18(6):1244–50.
13. Kim YS, Rhim H, Tae K, Park DW, Kim ST. Radiofrequency ablation of benign cold thyroid nodules: initial clinical experience. Thyroid. 2006;16(4):361–7.
14. Baek JH, Kim YS, Sung JY, Choi H, Lee JH. Locoregional control of metastatic well-differentiated thyroid cancer by ultrasound-guided radiofrequency ablation. AJR Am J Roentgenol. 2011;197(2):W331–6.
15. Deandrea M, Limone P, Basso E, Mormile A, Ragazzoni F, Gamarra E, et al. US-guided percutaneous radiofrequency thermal ablation for the treatment of solid benign hyperfunctioning or compressive thyroid nodules. Ultrasound Med Biol. 2008;34(5):784–91.
16. Spiezia S, Garberoglio R, Milone F, Ramundo V, Caiazzo C, Assanti AP, et al. Thyroid nodules and related symptoms are stably controlled two years after radiofrequency thermal ablation. Thyroid. 2009;19(3):219–25.
17. Sung JY, Baek JH, Kim YS, Jeong HJ, Kwak MS, Lee D, et al. One-step ethanol ablation of viscous cystic thyroid nodules. AJR Am J Roentgenol. 2008;191(6):1730–3.
18. Dupuy D, Monchik J, Decrea C, Pisharodi L. Radiofrequency ablation of regional recurrence from well-differentiated thyroid malignancy. Surgery. 2001;130:971–7.
19. Monchik JM, Donatini G, Iannuccilli J, Dupuy DE. Radiofrequency ablation and percutaneous ethanol injection treatment for recurrent local and distant well-differentiated thyroid carcinoma. Ann Surg. 2006;244(2):296–304.
20. Park KW, Shin JH, Han BK, Ko EY, Chung JH. Inoperable symptomatic recurrent thyroid cancers: preliminary result of radiofrequency ablation. Ann Surg Oncol. 2011;18(9):2564–8.
21. Carrafiello G, Lagana D, Mangini M, Dionigi G, Rovera F, Carcano G, et al. Treatment of secondary hyperparathyroidism with ultrasonographically guided percutaneous radiofrequency thermoablation. Surg Laparosc Endosc Percutan Tech. 2006;16(2):112–6.
22. Hansler J, Harsch IA, Strobel D, Hahn EG, Becker D. Treatment of a solitary adenoma of the parathyroid gland with ultrasound-guided percutaneous Radio-Frequency-Tissue-Ablation (RFTA). Ultraschall Med. 2002;23(3):202–6.
23. Cooper DS, Doherty GM, Haugen BR, Hauger BR, Kloos RT, Lee SL, et al. Revised American Thyroid Association management guidelines for patients with thyroid nodules and differentiated thyroid cancer. Thyroid. 2009;19(11):1167–214.
24. Gharib H, Papini E, Paschke R, Duick DS, Valcavi R, Hegedus L, et al. American Association of Clinical Endocrinologists, Associazione Medici Endocrinologi, and EuropeanThyroid Association Medical guidelines for clinical practice for the diagnosis and management of thyroid nodules. Endocr Pract. 2010;16 Suppl 1:1–43.
25. Jang SW, Baek JH, Kim JK, Sung JY, Choi H, Lim HK et al. How to manage the patients with unsatisfactory results after ethanol ablation for thyroid nodules: role of radiofrequency ablation. Eur J Radiol. 2011;81(5):905–910.
26. Ha EJ, Baek JH, Lee JH. The efficacy and complications of radiofrequency ablation of thyroid nodules. Curr Opin Endocrinol Diabetes Obes. 2011;18(5):310–4.
27. Pacella CM, Bizzarri G, Guglielmi R, Anelli V, Bianchini A, Crescenzi A, et al. Thyroid tissue: US-guided percutaneous interstitial laser ablation – a feasibility study. Radiology. 2000; 217(3):673–7.
28. Papini E, Guglielmi R, Bizzarri G, Graziano F, Bianchini A, Brufani C, et al. Treatment of benign cold thyroid nodules: a randomized clinical trial of percutaneous laser ablation versus levothyroxine therapy or follow-up. Thyroid. 2007;17(3):229–35.
29. Papini E, Guglielmi R, Bizzarri G, Pacella CM. Ultrasound-guided laser thermal ablation for treatment of benign thyroid nodules. Endocr Pract. 2004;10(3):276–83.
30. Valcavi R, Riganti F, Bertani A, Formisano D, Pacella CM. Percutaneous laser ablation of cold benign thyroid nodules: a 3-year follow-up study in 122 patients. Thyroid. 2010;20(11):1253–61.
31. Hegedus L. Therapy: a new nonsurgical therapy option for benign thyroid nodules? Nat Rev Endocrinol. 2009;5(9):476–8.

32. Esnault O, Franc B, Chapelon JY. Localized ablation of thyroid tissue by high-intensity focused ultrasound: improvement of noninvasive tissue necrosis methods. Thyroid. 2009; 19(10):1085–91.
33. Esnault O, Franc B, Monteil JP, Chapelon JY. High-intensity focused ultrasound for localized thyroid-tissue ablation: preliminary experimental animal study. Thyroid. 2004;14(12): 1072–6.
34. Esnault O, Rouxel A, Le Nestour E, Gheron G, Leenhardt L. Minimally invasive ablation of a toxic thyroid nodule by high-intensity focused ultrasound. AJNR Am J Neuroradiol. 2010; 31(10):1967–8.
35. Kovatcheva RD, Vlahov JD, Shinkov AD, Borissova AM, Hwang JH, Arnaud F, et al. High-intensity focused ultrasound to treat primary hyperparathyroidism: a feasibility study in four patients. AJR Am J Roentgenol. 2010;195(4):830–5.
36. Choi JW, Kwak S-H, Yoo SM, Song IS, Lee HY, Lee JB, et al. Ultrasound-guided radiofrequency ablation of thyroid gland: a preliminary study in dogs. J Korean Radiol Soc. 2005;52:333–41.

Chapter 8
Breast Ablation: Breast Carcinoma, Fibroadenomas

Rachel R. Bitton, Bruce L. Daniel, and Kim Butts Pauly

Standard Management of Breast Cancer

Standard management of breast cancer depends on the tumor type, biologic receptor status, and extent of disease (TNM staging). Detailed accepted treatment algorithms are available from the National Comprehensive Cancer Network [http://www.nccn.org] and are summarized here:

- Pure DCIS (Tis, N0, M0)

  - Mastectomy or breast conservation (lumpectomy & XRT; local control after lumpectomy requires tumor-free resection margins)
  - Systemic hormonal therapy considered for ER/PR-positive tumors treated with breast conservation

- Invasive breast carcinoma (IDC, ILC), <5 mm (T1a, N0, M0)

  - Mastectomy or breast conservation

- Invasive breast carcinoma (IDC, ILC), 5 mm–5 cm (T1b–T2, N0–1, M0)

  - Mastectomy or breast conservation
  - Adjuvant systemic therapy based on receptor status:

    ○ ER/PR positive: Hormonal therapy (e.g., tamoxifen or aromatase inhibitor) [some T1b–c, all T2].

R.R. Bitton, Ph.D. (✉) • K.B. Pauly, Ph.D.
Department of Radiology, Lucas Center for Imaging, Stanford University, School of Medicine, 1201 Welch Road, MC 5488, Stanford, CA 94305, USA
e-mail: rbitton@stanford.edu; kbpauly@stanford.edu

B.L. Daniel, M.D.
Department of Radiology, Stanford University, School of Medicine, 300 Pasteur Dr., H1307 MC 5621, Stanford, CA 94305, USA
e-mail: bdaniel@stanford.edu

T. Clark, T. Sabharwal (eds.), *Interventional Radiology Techniques in Ablation*, Techniques in Interventional Radiology, DOI 10.1007/978-0-85729-094-6_8, © Springer-Verlag London 2013

    ◦ Her2Neu positive: Cytotoxic therapy and trastuzumab [some T1b, most T1c, all T2].

    ◦ ER/PR negative and Her2Neu negative ("triple negative"): Cytotoxic therapy [some T1b, most T1c, all T2].

- Consider neoadjuvant therapy (before surgery) for large T2 tumors as a way to improve breast conservation.

• Invasive breast carcinoma (IDC, ILC), >5 cm (T3, N0–1, M0)

- Neoadjuvant chemotherapy (determined by receptor status) for:

    ◦ Locally inoperable tumors
    ◦ Large tumors as a potential way to enable breast conservation
    ◦ Rapidly growing tumors in patients needing urgent systemic therapy

- Mastectomy or breast conservation after successful neoadjuvant chemo
- Adjuvant systemic chemotherapy
- Possible chest wall irradiation

• Metastatic invasive breast cancer (IDC, ILC), any T, N2, M1

- Systemic chemotherapy determined by receptor status
- Post-chemo surgery and irradiation, determined by residual disease burden, for local control

Percutaneous tumor ablation provides less incremental benefit over surgery in the breast compared with many other organs:

• Breast surgery for early-stage tumors is fast, has low morbidity, and is frequently performed as an outpatient or "day-surgery" procedure.
• Modern "oncoplastic" surgery techniques for many tumors leave scars along the areolar margin where there is minimal cosmetic impact on the breast. This is especially true for smaller, centrally located tumors that are away from the skin and chest wall – the same tumors that could be considered candidates for ablation.
• Efficacy of surgery is easily assessed by histologically examining the inked margins of the excised tissue. Efficacy after ablation is assessed by imaging, which may be less accurate.
• Clinical studies for long-term follow-up results are still underway.
• Currently, there are no established, clinically accepted roles for image-guided breast cancer ablation.

Image-guided tumor ablation is being investigated in several scenarios:

• Salvage palliative therapy for local recurrences in patients who are not surgical candidates.
• Focal ablation of T1–T3 tumors with intent to provide better cosmetic outcome than lumpectomy (e.g., no skin scar).
• Focal ablation for palliation of benign fibroadenomas. Fibroadenoma (FA) is the most common benign breast mass. Clinically, fibroadenoma presents as a lump

and may be accompanied by pain. Fibroadenomas do not require treatment; however, palpable fibroadenomas distress some patients, who then request removal. The overall goal is to remove the palpable "lump" that causes anxiety or pain in some patients.

• Focal ablation prior to surgery to mark the extent of the target lesion, as a means of improving preoperative definition of disease compared with standard wire-localization methods.

Historically, minimally invasive image-guided breast tumor ablation has been performed with interstitial laser fibers, radiofrequency (RF) ablation probes, cryoprobes, and external high-intensity focused ultrasound, using ultrasound, CT, or MRI for guidance. A summary of clinically relevant studies in breast ablation is given in Table 8.1.

These procedures are typically done on an outpatient basis, commonly using no more than local anesthesia, such as local lidocaine injections in probe-based ablations, and/or conscious sedation. Posttreatment, contrast-enhanced MRI has shown good agreement in assessment of ablation margins when compared with histological results but may be difficult in cases with non-enhancing DCIS where MRI does not adequately define the tumor margins. A comparison for each ablation technique presented in this chapter is given in Table 8.2.

Probe-Based Ablations

Image guidance in probe-based ablations has been mostly ultrasound, although cryoablation, RF, and laser ablation have all reported breast interventions using MR guidance and MR thermometry. Probe placement can pose a significant challenge in conventional closed-bore MRI, where access to breast is limited during imaging.

Probe placement has been investigated either by freehand methods or varying degrees of breast stabilization ranging from light stabilization (breast MRI coil) to firm (compression plates) stabilization. Firm stabilization using stereotactic positioners combined with compression plates has been used to facilitate needle and probe placement; however, lesions may still move under the force of the advancing needle, as seen commonly with X-ray-guided procedures under firm compression. Other challenges associated with compression plates include potentially limited access to the anterior breast or the posterior breast/axillary tail [1] and in ultrasound-guided interventions, the requirement of an acoustic window for coupling. Since excessive breast compression has been shown to interfere with MRI lesion enhancement [2], light stabilization has been recommended for MR-guided probe-based breast interventions [3].

The heating phase of probe-based ablations has predominately been monitored via ultrasound, where observations of hyperechoic regions indicate heated tissue. Additional ablation indicators used include temperature measurements from thermocouples inserted adjacent to the ablation site and impedance measurements, in the case of RF ablation. Although ultrasound provides real-time treatment monitoring, inaccurate visualization of ablation margins due to the large hypoechoic regions surrounding heated tissue has been reported [4, 5].

Table 8.1 Summary of breast ablation clinical trials

	No. of patients	Image guidance/methods	Tumor characteristics	Complete ablation/endpoint	Complications/cause of failures
Cryoablation					
Sabel [16]	27	Ultrasound Double freeze/thaw	δ 2.0 cm ultrasound visible primary invasive	78 %	None reported/noncalcified DCIS
Morin [10]	25	MRI	<7.0 cm Proven invasive carcinoma	52 %	Skin burn at probe entry
Roubidoux [15]	9	Ultrasound	<1.8 cm Proven invasive ductal and colloid carcinoma	78 %	None reported
Pusztaszeri [13]	11	MRI	<2.0 cm Proven invasive	36 %	Skin ulceration (45 %)
Manenti [17]	15	Ultrasound Double freeze/thaw	<1 cm Proven T1 invasive US and MRI visible	93 %	Nodular thickening (6 %)
Littrup [12]	42	Ultrasound Double freeze/passive, active thaw	Biopsy-proven *fibroadenoma*, mean 4.2 cm	N/A US size reduction of 73 %	None reported
RFA					
Jeffrey [20]	5	Ultrasound Array – 2 cycle	>5.0 cm Proven T3–T4	80 %	None reported
Izzo [4]	26	Ultrasound Array – 2 cycle	0.7–3.0 cm Proven T1–T2 invasive	96 %	Full-thickness skin burn (4 %)
Burak [5]	10	Ultrasound DCE MRI eval. Array – 2 cycle	0.8–1.6 cm Proven T1 invasive	89 %	Minimal breast ecchymosis (10 %)

Earashi [21]	24	Stereotactic (4 %) ultrasound (96 %) Array – 1 cycle	0.5–2.4 cm invasive and noninvasive ductal carcinoma	100 %	None reported
Imoto [24]	30	Ultrasound Array – 2 cycle	0.9–2.4 cm Proven T1N0	92 %	Skin burn (7 %) Muscle burn (23 %)
Medina-Franco [26]	25	Ultrasound Saline-cooled tip – 3 cycle	0.9–3.8 cm Proven T1–T2 invasive	76 %	None reported
Kinoshita [29]	49	Ultrasound Saline-cooled tip general anesthesia	0.5–3.0 cm proven T1–T2 invasive	61 %	Skin burn (4 %) Muscle burn (6 %)
Microwave					
Gardner [35]	10	Ultrasound Dual probe array	1.0–8.0 cm Proven T1–T3 invasive	0 %	Skin burn Skin flap necrosis
Dooley [39]	34	Ultrasound Dual probe array MWA+chemotherapy	1.7 mean Proven T1–T2 invasive	6 %	Skin burns (8 %) Erythema (12 %) Intolerable discomfort (14.7 %)
Vargas [37]	25	Ultrasound Dual probe array	Proven T1–T2 invasive	8 %	Skin burn Erythema
Zhou [41]	41	Ultrasound 2.5-GHz probe	<3.0 cm Proven T1–T2 unifocal	90 %	Skin burn
Laser					
Mumtaz [49]	20	MRI	2.2 cm mean Proven T1–T4	None reported	None reported
Akimov [43]	35	Ultrasound	b.–6.0 cm Proven T1–T3 invasive	Unclear	Gaseous rupture of tumor
Dowlatshahi [45]	54	Stereotactic Ultrasound	0.5–2.3 cm Proven T1–T2 invasive	70 %	Small skin burns
Van Esser [51]	14	Ultrasound	0.8–3.7 cm Unifocal invasive	50 %	Skin burn, pneumothorax

Table 8.1 (continued)

	No. of patients	Image guidance/methods	Tumor characteristics	Complete ablation/endpoint	Complications/cause of failures
HIFU					
Hynynen [61]	19	MRI + thermometry	Biopsy-proven *fibroadenoma* 0.7–6.5 cm^3	N/A 73 % response in postcontrast T1w images	Transient edema in pectoralis muscle (5 %)
Gianfelice [63]	12	MRI + thermometry "Mark 2" protocol	<3.5 cm Invasive lobular (11 %) Invasive ductal carcinoma (89 %)	24 %	2nd-degree skin burns (17 %)
Gianfelice [67]	24	MRI No resection 1–2 FUS sessions	0.6–2.5 cm Proven T1–T2 invasive	79 % negative biopsy at 6 and 7 months	2nd-degree skin burn (4 %)
Zippel [68]	10	MRI + unclear	<3.0 cm Proven T1–T2 invasive	20 %	Pain (10 %), 2nd-degree skin burn (10 %)
Furusawa [62]	30	MRI + thermometry	δ 2.5 cm Proven T1–T2 invasive	53.5 %	Skin burn (3 %)
Wu [64]	23	Ultrasound	δ 6.0 cm Proven T1–T2 invasive	100 %	Skin burn (4 %), moderate pain (17 %), sensation of heaviness (4 %)

Table 8.2 Comparison of breast ablation techniques

	Probes	Complete ablation rates (%)	Advantages	Limitations/restrictions	Number of published clinical studies
MWA	Probe antenna/ antenna array	0–90	Less susceptible to perivascular heat sinks. Theoretical preferential heating of carcinoma due to elevated water content	Heating profile varies dependent upon tissue water content. Elliptically shaped ablations	Very little
Laser	Optical fiber with saline drip	13–76	Compatible with MR thermometry	Laser tip sensitive to thermal damage. Small ablation zone, multiple fibers needed for large volume tumors	Moderate
RFA	Single-tip electrode or umbrella electrode array	76–100	Large ablation volumes possible with scaled arrays	Requires ground pads. Dessication of tissue near probe limits heat conduction and ablation of large tumor volume	Considerable
Cryo	Single probe 2.4– 2.7 mm diameter	36–52	Cooling may provide local analgesic effects during treatment	Elliptically shaped iceball formation. Low complete ablation rates	Moderate
HIFU	None	20–100	Noninvasive. Compatible with MRI guidance (without probe artifact) and MR thermometry for temperature monitoring	Multiple sequential lesions required to ablate tumor volume. Long treatment time for large tumor volumes. Significant local anesthetic and conscious sedation is required	Moderate

Cryoablation

Cryosurgery of breast cancer was reported at least as early as the mid-1800s by James Arnott [6]. Prior to imaging guidance, cryosurgery has been used primarily for nonoperative patients, including those with locally advanced disease, or recurrences [7].

Image guidance for breast cryosurgery has primarily used ultrasound. Ultrasound-guided open probe placement was reported in 1985 [8]. Minimally invasive ultrasound-guided cryosurgery was reported in 1997 [9].

Shadowing from the edge of the developing iceball limits sonographic monitoring of freezing. MRI [10] and CT [11] have both been reported as alternative methods to fully image the iceball in breast tissue in 3 dimensions.

Procedure

Patients are prepped and draped in typical sterile fashion. The breast tumor location is identified by quadrant via ultrasound or other imaging modality. Protocols report injecting the skin overlying the tumor and the projected probe path to the tumor with buffered lidocaine solutions. This was followed by a skin incision of 3 mm prior to probe insertion. Single 1.4–2.7-mm-diameter cryoprobe placement has been placed at, or just beyond, the distal margin of the tumor, as seen on imaging (Fig. 8.1). This technique is intended to provide equal treatment on both sides of the tumor in the longitudinal plane of the freeze zone, since iceball formation may present as an elliptical shape which tracks slightly along the probe shaft. Alternatively, multiple probes may be used to freeze larger or more irregularly shaped targets. Probes have been placed directly, or initiated with a trocar needle whose stylet is removed and replaced with the cryoprobe. In that case, the coaxial sheath was retracted slightly from the probe tip and used to insulate the insertion tract from freezing. Some devices have a vacuum-insulated trocar tip integrated into the probe. In order to fix probe placement, a short, low duty cycle activation of the system to create a "stick freeze" has been reported. Iceball formation has been investigated under single freeze and multiple freeze protocols of decreasing duty cycle. Periodic saline injections between the tumor and the skin surface or chest wall have been used to maintain safe boundaries of the advancing iceball. A low duty cycle active thaw facilitates probe removal. Manual pressure of up to 20 min to prevent hematoma formation has been reported [12].

Cryoablation for Breast Cancer

- Results from 5 "treat and resect" studies show variable efficacy for cryosurgery from 36 to 83 % compared with subsequent excision [13–15]. The highest complete ablation rates occurred in tumors <1 cm [16, 17].
- Failures attributed to large lesion size (diameter >15 mm), *DCIS*, and poor quality imaging.
- Ongoing study *without resection* shows no local recurrences among 22 sites in 11 patients with an average follow-up of 18 months [11].
- Multiple probes facilitate treatment of larger and irregular lesions.
- Performed with local anesthesia only. Saline injections/warming bags have been used to protect the skin from freezing.
- Localized analgesic effects during the freeze cycle have been reported [17].

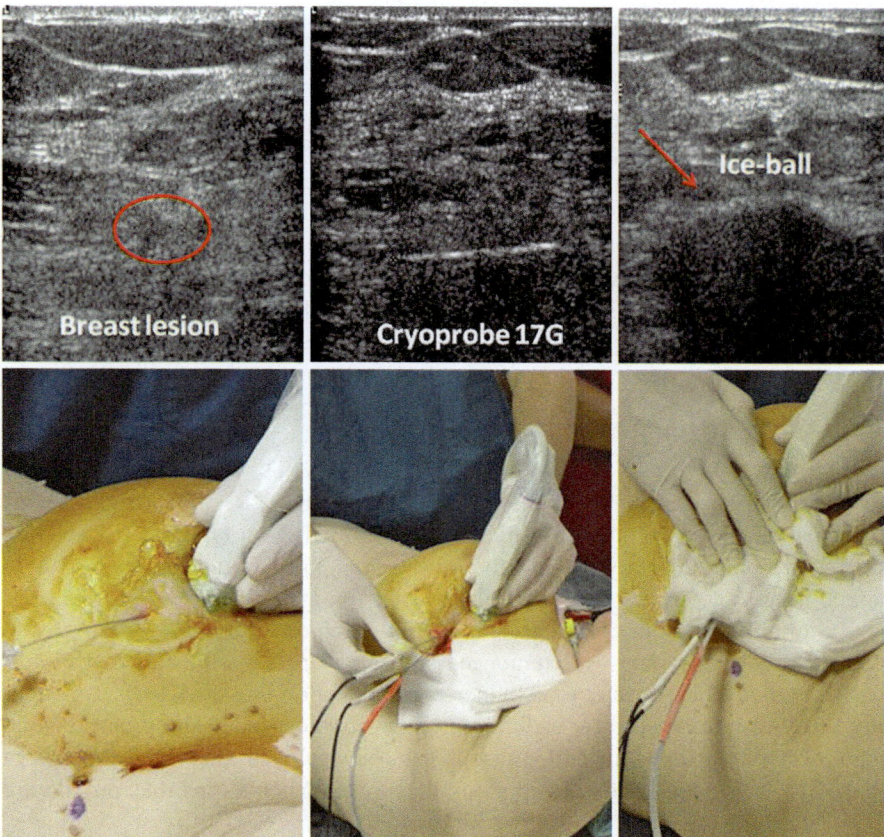

Fig. 8.1 Cryoablation procedure. The devices were placed percutaneously by ultrasound guidance using an ultrasound probe at 5–12 MHz. After skin incision with a scalpel (3 mm), the cryoprobe (17 G isotherms) and two thermocouples for temperature monitoring were positioned. The compressed argon gas passes through the needle during cryoablation, cooling the tip and generating the iceball in the adjacent tissue because of adiabatic effect (Joule–Thompson phenomenon). The compressed helium gas expanding in the coaxial needle heats the exposed tip of the probe arresting the progression of the procedure and/or alternatively dissolving the iceball at the end of the second cooling cycle by restoring the electrode–tissue interface. The application of hot patches on the skin adjacent to the probe has also significantly reduced the after treatment skin rashes incidence by achieving a good definitive cosmetics [17] (*Reprinted from* Manenti et al. [17], with permission from Springer)

Cryoablation for Fibroadenomas

- "Ultrasound-guided FA cryoablation has been widely studied [12, 18]. Tumors ≤2 cm in diameter are more likely to become non-palpable, but involution often takes 6–12 months, or longer.
- Fibroadenoma cryoablation is frequently performed in the office setting.

Cryoablation for Preoperative Lesion Marking

- Non-palpable tumors that are found by imaging must be marked preoperatively using imaging in order for surgeons to excise them.
- Cryoprobe(s) are placed into the mass sonographically at the start of surgery.
- Freezing creates a palpable mass, which is then used by surgeons to remove the mass.
- Single randomized controlled trial showed similar tumor margin control compared with standard wire localization and reported that cryo-assisted lumpectomy enabled slightly smaller resection specimens [19].

Radio Frequency Ablation

Of the probe-based ablation techniques for breast cancer, RF ablation (RFA) has the most extensive volume of clinical work reported. Two types of RF ablation probes are predominately used in the breast: array probes and internally cooled single-needle electrodes. The umbrella-shaped tines of RF array probes vary in size and number of tines. The probe is often chosen dependent on lesion size, so that the prongs encompass the tumor mass. Cooled single-needle electrodes internally circulate chilled water to help increase conduction into the tissues surrounding the active probe surface, enabling a larger ablation zone. The probes can be equipped with a retractable thermocouple to be deployed after the needle is in place, or integrated with the tip(s) of the probe. MRI-compatible probes are available.

Procedure

Using image guidance, the RF array probe is placed in the center of the lesion, where the tines of the electrode array are deployed. After the treatment is complete, the tines are retracted back into the needle, and the probe is removed. The current induced in RFA requires a return current path. Grounding pads applied to the skin's surface are used to complete the path; they can be placed on each thigh.

There is no widely accepted consensus on the protocol of RFA in the breast. Typically, probe impedance and power level are treatment progress/completion indicators. However, in the breast, there is added complexity due to tissue heterogeneity. The widely variable proportions of fat and fibroglandular tissue can result in an inhomogeneous conductivity profile.

Some procedure complications include entry site burns, ablation zone skin burns (particularly in patients with small breasts), and skin burns at the grounding pads. Pad burns are preventable by using adhesion tape to ensure tension is taken off the wires, so that the entire pad surface is in contact with the skin, or by using multiple pads.

RFA in Breast Cancer

- Several groups followed the first pilot study of RFA in breast cancer by Jeffery et al. in 1999 [20] with feasibility studies for small breast cancer [5, 21–27].
- Treatment protocols consisting of a two-phase cycle have been reported [4, 5, 24]. In this protocol, base powers of 5–10 W are applied for 2 min, followed by 2–5 W increments until the tissue impedance rises rapidly, and power roll-off is seen, which indicates tissue coagulation. After a brief cooling period, a second cycle of heating is applied with the same incremental protocol.
- As a method of protecting the overlying skin and pectoralis major muscle from RFA-induced burns, some groups used a 20–40 ml of 5 % glucose injection in the subdermal tissues and retromammary spaces [21, 24, 28].
- A phase II trial, which looked at the safety and efficacy using a saline cooled single-tip electrode, showed a 92 % complete ablation rate and low (3 %) complication rate [26], while Kinoshita et al. reported a 61 % complete ablation rate [29].
- Debulking of large tumors was studied in nine patients with either stage IIIA, IIIB, and stage IV cancer followed by mastectomy [30]. Using an 8-MHz probe and continuous saline injection to the tumor site, significant reduction in tumor size was reported: initial mean tumor size 122.1 ± 71.5 cm^3, postablation mean tumor size 82.2 ± 63.4 cm^3, as measured by ultrasound.
- Three studies did not use a "treat and resect" protocol. In these protocols, clinical and imaging follow-up was planned in lieu of postablation surgery.

  - Two of these were in elderly inoperable patients [31, 32].
  - The third study used general anesthesia for the procedure, followed by postablation biopsy and adjuvant radiotherapy [28]. No viable tumor tissue was found in biopsy NADH–diaphorase staining in 24 of 29 patients; however, long-term follow-up results are not yet available from this study. Complications included a 3rd-degree skin burn and a patient who developed chronic granulomatous mastitis.
  - In a 52-patient study where RFA was accompanied by adjuvant chemo- and/ or endocrine-therapy and radiotherapy, no recurrences were found on a 15-month (average) follow-up. However, no long-term follow-up results have been reported [27].

- Some study contraindications have been listed as: diffuse calcification according to mammography, multifocal carcinoma, and evidence of extensive intraductal components on magnetic resonance (MR) mammography [21, 24].

RFA in Fibroadenoma

- Treatment of fibroadenoma with RFA is extremely limited. In a letter to the editor, a short report of two patients with a fibroadenoma ranging from 1.8 to 3.0 cm were treated with an array probe in a 2-cycle protocol [33]. Both patients reported palpable indurations over the ablation site that subsided over a 6-month period.

Microwave Ablation

Microwave ablation (MWA) in the breast involves placement of a needle electrode probe directly into the target tumor. The probe acts as an antenna, generating microwaves between 900 MHz and 2.45 GHz selectively agitating water molecules to a critical point. The oscillation of the water molecules generates friction, and heat from this process creates the thermal ablation. Unlike RFA, the method does not require patient grounding pads.

MWA image guidance in all reported and ongoing clinical trials in the breast is exclusively guided by ultrasound with reports of a hyperechoic region surrounding the probe [34].

The FDA-approved device in the initial breast trials included a 915-MHz MWA array in which a pair of catheter-based probes was inserted into the compressed breast opposite each other to create a central focus within the tumor [35]. Unlike the retractable prongs used in RFA, the needle tip probe ablation lesion tends to be more elliptical. The expected short-axis diameter measures slightly greater than 2 cm. Multiple probes or sessions may be needed to treat large tumors.

Procedure

The patient is typically positioned prone, the breast placed through a hole in the treatment table, then compressed to a thickness of roughly 4–8 cm dependent on breast size. To prevent skin burns, compression plates and airflow techniques (including auxiliary fans) are applied to the skin to cool the breast during treatment [35]. A window in the compression plates allows probe insertion and ultrasound image guidance. Temperature probes can be inserted via catheter to measure surrounding tumor temperature. Additional temperature probes have been taped to the skin and nipple to monitor skin temperature during therapy. Treatment completion has been determined by desired thermal dose, calculated from external and internal temperature probes over time.

Microwave Ablation in Breast Cancer

- One of the proposed advantages for microwave therapy in breast cancer is that microwave (like RF) preferentially heats high-water, high-ion content tissues. Since breast carcinomas are reported to often have a higher water content than fatty tissue and normal fibroglandular tissue [36], microwave energy could be preferential to breast carcinoma by heating it faster than surrounding healthy tissue.
- Clinical trials using MWA in the breast have been limited compared with other ablative techniques. Four completed trials involving invasive carcinoma of the breast have been reported by the same group [35, 37–39]. The first reported trial was a phase I safety trial of ten patients with biopsy-proven invasive carcinoma who received MWA prior to mastectomy. Reduction in tumor size, a skin burn, and a skin

flap necrosis were reported with no results of complete tumor ablation. A phase II dose escalation study in 2004 (based on the phase I safety trial) showed 2 out of 25 patients with complete tumor ablation as confirmed by H&E staining [37].

- Randomized study for early-stage carcinoma, MWA compared to surgery alone, treated tumors between 0.7 and 3.6 cm with treatment times between 140 and 210 min; the desired peak temperature of >48 °C was achieved in (44.1 %) patients, hematoma/seroma reported in 17.6 % of patients. Although results showed reduced positive tumor margins of the MWA-treated tumors (0 %) compared with surgery alone (9.8 %), no statistical significance resulted from the difference. Exclusion criteria reported patients with extensive DCIS [34].

- A cohort study evaluated the ability to perform sentinel node biopsy after a microwave ablation of breast cancer. Sentinel lymph node mapping was successful in 19 of 21 patients (91 %) [40].

- Recent study of US-guided MWA, operating at a higher frequency of 2.4 GHz and using general anesthesia, was followed by mastectomy. It showed complete coagulation in 95 % (36 of 38) of patients with small invasive cancers, with a low rate of 33 % (1 of 3) in patients with DCIS. The mean ablation volumes were 2.77×2.06 cm, with only minor complications reported [41].

Laser Ablation

Laser ablation (LA) has also been referred to as laser-induced interstitial thermotherapy (LIIT) or laser-induced thermotherapy or interstitial laser therapy; for brevity, this chapter uses LA.

Although Nd:YAG lasers have been evaluated for thermal ablation in the breast [42], diode lasers are predominately used, they provide greater portability, and deliver lower energy levels (2–10 W) over a longer time (10–30 min), which are better suited for controlled tumor ablation [43–46]. The size of tumor destruction can be increased with the use of several fibers. Laser treatments may be performed under imaging guidance (mammography, ultrasound, or MRI). A target temperature of >60 °C is commonly reached [47].

Initial findings in LA reported a reduction in ablation efficiency due to damage of the fiber tip by high ablative temperatures. Dowlatshahi et al. proposed a para-axial saline drip delivered to the fiber tip to prevent damage, currently used on FDA-approved devices [45].

Macroscopically, LA-ablated tissue appears as concentric rings. The central cavity is surrounded by what is referred to as a "pale zone," associated with liponecrosis, peripheral hemorrhages, and other nonviable zones. It is suggested by some investigators that the outer rim represents the margins of cancer destruction [47].

Traditional ultrasound image guidance and monitoring of heated zone is common; however, several groups have reported the use of MR guidance and monitoring [48, 49]. LA is well suited for MR guidance and monitoring since the laser fiber does not produce the metal image artifact possibly seen with RF and microwave probes.

Procedure

A breast stereotactic device and insertion of two probes, the optical fiber for ablation, and the temperature probe have been used. Depending on the size of the optical
fiber, 14–17-gauge needles placed the optical fiber in the center of the tumor,
confirmed by imaging. The needle is then retracted to avoid heat conduction to the
skin, and in the case of para-axial drip devices, a pump attached to the probe is used
to continuously irrigate the laser fiber tip with saline during the treatment. The adjacent thermal probe continuously measures local temperature, where 50–60 °C
threshold temperatures of peripheral sensors in the breast tissue have been used as
the indicator for treatment completion [50].

LA in Treatment of Breast Cancer

- Trials have reported a range of 13–76 % complete ablation for patients with
  T1–T3 tumors [45, 46].
- LA procedure complications are predominantly small skin burns; however, pneumothorax and a gaseous rupture of the tumor were reported as a serious complication [43, 51].
- While no significant correlation between margin of necrosed tissue has been
  reported on ultrasound and mammography, contrast-enhanced MRI has shown
  good correlation in the hypointense regions defining the extent of LA necrosis
  and residual tumor [49, 52].

Laser Ablation for Fibroadenomas

- There is an ongoing multicenter clinical trial of ablation of biopsy-proven
  fibroadenomas under ultrasound guidance with local anesthesia [53].
- Inclusion criteria: Fibroadenomas not exceeding 2 cm that are mammo and ultrasound visible, minimum of 0.5 cm away from the skin and chest wall.
- Ablation and laser probes inserted via 14-gauge needles, the ablation laser probe,
  and the temperature probe placed adjacent to the laser probe.
- Typical ablation time is 15–30 min for lesions under 2 cm.
- Exclusion criteria: Phyllodes, atypia, and equivocal pathology report. Long-term
  follow-up from a 2-patient laser ablation study reported shrinkage 40 and 50 %
  at 8- and 6-year follow-up, respectively [50].

Focused Ultrasound Ablations

The use of focused ultrasound (FUS) or high-intensity focused ultrasound (HIFU)
in tissue ablation was reported as early as 1942, where lesions were formed in liver
and brain tissue [54]. FUS does not require percutaneous access to the breast and
may offer a more favorable cosmetic result over incision-type probe ablations.

MR Guidance

In general, FUS is well suited to MR guidance because real-time imaging, like ultrasound, is not needed to guide placement of a probe. FUS ablations in the breast are increasingly utilizing MR guidance for its high sensitivity, tumor margin accuracy, and ability to assess postprocedural ablation margins [55–57]. MR thermometry using the proton-resonance frequency (PRF) shift method is a widely accepted tool to monitor temperature in ablation targets such as the liver and uterine fibroids. It has been used in clinical breast ablation trials to monitor temperature within the tumor [58]. However, it is currently unreliable in adipose and mixed adipose/fibroglandular tissue found in the breast. T1-weighted images can be used to qualitatively show heating, since heat lengthens the T1 of both fibroglandular and adipose tissues, causing signal loss on T1-weighted images. MR-guided FUS clinical trials have used MR thermometry to monitor temperature within the tumor boundary, although alternative approaches to temperature monitoring in adipose tissue have been proposed [59, 60]. The first report of multipatient clinical MR-guided FUS in the breast was in the ablation of fibroadenomas [61]. MRI contrast-enhanced images show a breast carcinoma tumor before and after MR–FUS ablation (Fig. 8.2). Note the normal rim of enhancement around the ablation due to local hyperemia.

Procedure

In many of the published trials, mammography, ultrasound, and core biopsy are followed by pre- and postprocedural contrast-enhanced MRI using T1-weighted 3D gradient echo and T2-weighted fast spin echo imaging with fat saturation for tumor evaluation.

Patient Preparation

Adequate acoustic coupling to the skin, using gel or water, is paramount in the prevention of skin burns. Margins of safety for focused ultrasound ablation are determined by the tumor–skin distance and tumor–chest wall distance. These are in place to protect against skin burns and unwanted heating near the chest wall due to increased absorption of ultrasound energy in bone/muscle tissue.
MR-Guided FUS
- Patients have been positioned prone, with the breast situated in a special MR FUS breast coil.
- The transducer faced upward toward the chest wall and was coupled to the skin with an acoustically transparent gel pad and/or water bath.
- Local anesthesia including 2 % injection of mepivacaine behind the tumor was used prior to ablation [62].
- Studies have used analgesic combined with a sedative prior to treatment to reduce anxiety and unnecessary motion [63].

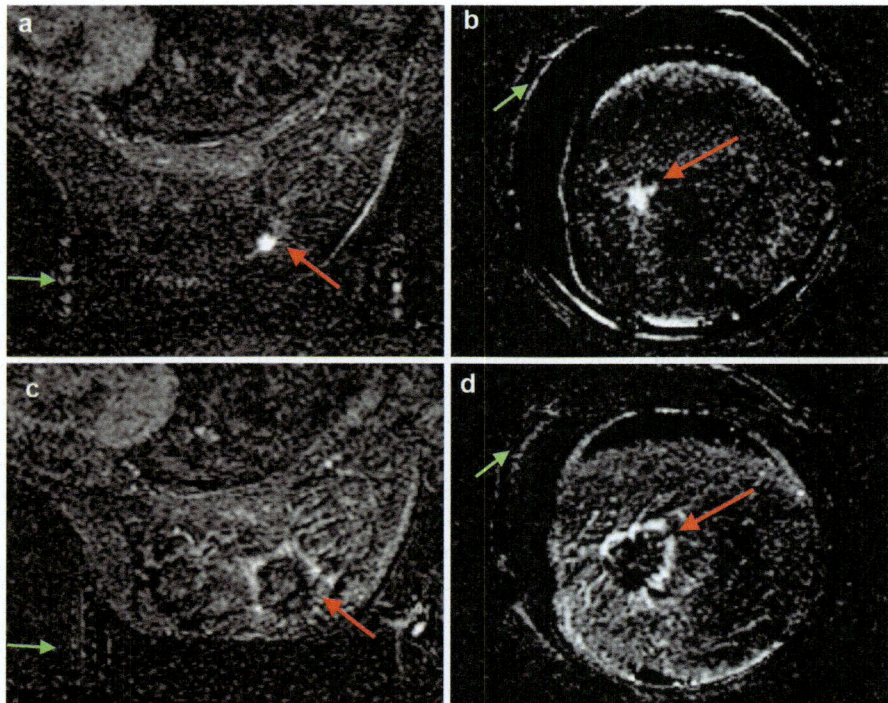

Fig. 8.2 Contrast-enhanced breast MRI with transducer present (**a**) and (**b**) before MR–FUS ablation (axial, coronal) and (**c**) and (**d**) after MR–FUS ablation. *Red arrows* point to the tumor location pretreatment and the ablated zone posttreatment. *Green arrows* point to the ultrasonic transducer (Images courtesy Dr. Hidemi Furusawa, furusawa@breastopia.org)

Ultrasound-Guided FUS
- Patients treated with ultrasound guidance were positioned prone, the breast placed in a water bath.
- An integrated probe with a 3D imaging (3.5–5 MHz) and therapy (1.6 MHz) was submerged in the bath facing the breast.
- General anesthesia and associated monitoring (blood pressure, respiration, etc.) has been used in a portion of patients (19 of 23 patients) [64].

Planning and Treatment

In the ultrasound-guided system, the treatment focal location was assumed to be the center of the ultrasound image, since both imaging and therapy transducers were designed to converge to the same spot. In MR-guided systems, calibration is performed using a low-power sonication that induces a few degree temperature rise, allowing the focal spot to be directly visualized by either changes in T1 or thermometry.

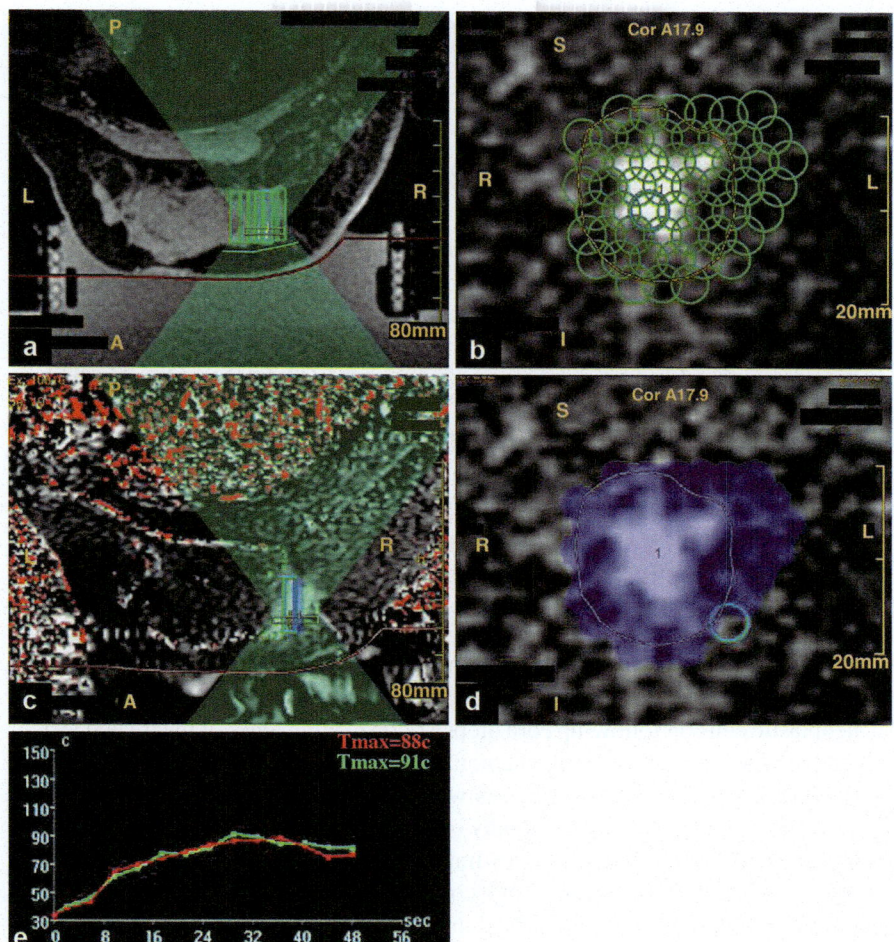

Fig. 8.3 MR–FUS interface shows (**a**) axial MRI showing overlay of planned ablation spots (*green rectangles*), ultrasound beam path (*green*), and skin line (*red*). (**b**) Coronal view of planned ablation spots (*green circles*) around the contrasted enhanced tumor. Note the sonications extend beyond the tumor boundary. (**c**) MR thermometry image during treatment. The *yellow cross* indicates the location of temperature measurement over the treatment time shown in (**e**). (**d**) Coronal view of breast with overlay of posttreatment thermal dose (*purple*). *Green circle* indicates next sonication (Images courtesy Dr. Hidemi Furusawa, furusawa@breastopia.org)

FUS lesions are elliptically shaped. Large ablation volumes are achieved by a succession of overlapping sonications. Figure 8.3 shows an example of a breast treatment, including planning and heating images. The region of treatment and individual ablations are generally prescribed on planning images. The transducer is mechanically and/or electronically steered sequentially to each ablation location. There is no clear agreement in the literature on sonication power and sonication duration for breast ablation. Treatment power has been reported as focal peak intensities, ranging from 500 to 15,000 W/cm^2.

Focused Ultrasound for Breast Cancer

- The first case of MR-guided FUS to treat breast cancer was reported by Huber et al. [65]. Following a series of sheep ablations, one patient with biopsy-proven breast cancer was treated with FUS using no anesthetic. Both MR thermometry and T2-weighted images between ultrasound pulses were used for monitoring. Five days after the ablation, the patient received BCS, adjuvant local radiotherapy, and tamoxifen. Partial necrosis of the tumor was reported.
- In a 30-patient trial using MR-guided FUS for biopsy-proven cases, 15 (53.5 %) of 28 had 100 % necrosis of the ablated tumor, 10 (35.8 %) had 95–97 %, and 3 (10.7 %) had less than 95 % necrosis [62].
- A randomized phase II trial using ultrasound-guided ablation found 100 % complete ablation by using wide "surgical" ablation margins of 1.5–2.2 cm beyond the extent of the tumor, into normal tissue. Nineteen of the 23 patients were treated using general anesthesia [66].
- MR-guided FUS was added as an adjunctive therapy in patients who were poor candidates for surgical resection. Success was defined as the absence of viable neoplastic cells on follow-up core biopsy of up to eight areas of the treated lesion. All patients were treated with chemotherapy prior to FUS [67].
- Exclusion criteria reported: patients whose lesions were outside the margins of safety for US ablation consisted only of microcalcifications [67], patients receiving anticoagulation therapy, breast implants, inability to tolerate prone position for extended period of time, and conventional MR contraindications (metal implants, claustrophobia, etc.) [68].

Focused Ultrasound for Fibroadenomas

- Eleven fibroadenomas in 19 patients were treated with MR-guided FUS using local anesthesia and contrast T1-weighted images. Three of 11 lesions showed no decrease in posttreatment contrast uptake. Potential causes for lack of ablation were patient motion and low acoustic power (ultrasound energy and imaging sequences were not fixed patient to patient) [61].

Focused Ultrasound for Preoperative Lesion Marking

- Hyperthermic breast tumor volume ablations including RF ablation and FUS, have reported an increase in postablation breast tissue stiffness upon gross examination, although the change in palpability was not quantified [20, 33, 64, 69].

- Recent preliminary studies have proposed the use of MR-guided FUS for lesion marking by creating FUS ablations around a non-palpable tumor perimeter. The FUS lesions create a palpable border, for potential use as a surgical guide of tumor location and shape [70, 71].

Additional Considerations

- Greatest success in published breast tumor ablations appears to be in smaller (T1–T2) primary unifocal tumors.
- Ablative treatments are not recommended for tumors that do not have well-demarcated boundaries visible on ultrasound or MRI. This may include multifocal invasive lobular carcinoma, DCIS, and mucinous colloid carcinoma, where cases of poorly defined borders and underestimation of margins have been reported [72].
- All prognostic tumor histopathologic characteristics such as mitotic index, histological grade, and ER/PR/HER-2 status should be firmly established by biopsy prior to ablative treatment. Thus, the biopsy needle must be large enough to allow for such a sample (14 gauge or larger has been reported).
- There is no protocol across studies for systematic and accurate histopathologic assessment of tumor cell viability. Across studies, there is variance in the time between tumor ablation and surgical resection. Protocols range from surgical resection immediately following ablation to 56 days postablation [44, 45]. In addition, commonly used H&E stains are not ideal since proliferation markers may remain positive even after ablation. Some groups have shifted to use NADH staining, which is more accurate although perhaps impractical in the clinical setting, as it requires samples be snap frozen of before they are fixed [51]. These variations affect the statistics of complete ablation rates.
- It is not clear if lymph drainage is disrupted from local ablation treatment. Although studies have reported SNB both before and after treatment, SNB timing may be theoretically more reliable prior to ablative treatment.

References

1. Daniel BL, Butts K, Glover GH, Cooper C, Herfkens RJ. Breast cancer: gadolinium-enhanced MR imaging with a 0.5-T open imager and three-point Dixon technique. Radiology. 1998;207(1):183–90.
2. Kuhl CK, Elevelt A, Leutner CC, Gieseke J, Pakos E, Schild HH. Interventional breast MR imaging: clinical use of a stereotactic localization and biopsy device. Radiology. 1997;204(3):667–75.
3. Daniel BL. Intraprocedural magnetic resonance imaging-guided interventions in the breast. Top Magn Reson Imaging. 2000;11(3):184–90.
4. Izzo F, Thomas R, Delrio P, Rinaldo M, Vallone P, DeChiara A, et al. Radiofrequency ablation in patients with primary breast carcinoma: a pilot study in 26 patients. Cancer. 2001;92(8):2036–44.
5. Burak WE, Agnese DM, Povoski SP, Yanssens TL, Bloom KJ, Wakely PE, et al. Radiofrequency ablation of invasive breast carcinoma followed by delayed surgical excision. Cancer. 2003;98(7):1369–76.

6. Cooper SM, Dawber RP. The history of cryosurgery. J R Soc Med. 2001;94(4):196–201.
7. Ablin RJ. The use of cryosurgery for breast cancer. Arch Surg. 1998;133(1):106.
8. Rand RW, Rand RP, Eggerding FA, Field M, Denbesten L, King W, et al. Cryolumpectomy for breast cancer: an experimental study. Cryobiology. 1985;22(4):307–18.
9. Staren ED, Sabel MS, Gianakakis LM, Wiener GA, Hart VM, Gorski M, et al. Cryosurgery of breast cancer. Arch Surg. 1997;132(1):28–33; discussion 34.
10. Morin J, Traoré A, Dionne G, Dumont M, Fouquette B, Dufour M, et al. Magnetic resonance-guided percutaneous cryosurgery of breast carcinoma: technique and early clinical results. Can J Surg. 2004;47(5):347–51.
11. Littrup PJ, Jallad B, Chandiwala-Mody P, D'Agostini M, Adam BA, Bouwman D. Cryotherapy for breast cancer: a feasibility study without excision. J Vasc Interv Radiol. 2009;20(10):1329–41.
12. Littrup PJ, Freeman-Gibb L, Andea A, White M, Amerikia KC, Bouwman D, et al. Cryotherapy for breast fibroadenomas. Radiology. 2005;234(1):63–72.
13. Pusztaszeri M, Vlastos G, Kinkel K, Pelte M-F. Histopathological study of breast cancer and normal breast tissue after magnetic resonance-guided cryotherapy ablation. Cryobiology. 2007;55(1):44–51.
14. Zhao Z, Wu F. Minimally-invasive thermal ablation of early-stage breast cancer: a systemic review. Eur J Surg Oncol. 2010;36(12):1149–55.
15. Roubidoux MA, Sabel MS, Bailey JE, Kleer CG, Klein KA, Helvie MA. Small (<2.0 cm) breast cancers: mammographic and US findings at US-guided cryoablation - initial experience. Radiology. 2004;233(3):857–67.
16. Sabel MS, Kaufman CS, Whitworth P, Chang H, Stocks LH, Simmons R, et al. Cryoablation of early-stage breast cancer: work-in-progress report of a multi-institutional trial. Ann Surg Oncol. 2004;11(5):542–9.
17. Manenti G, Perretta T, Gaspari E, Pistolese CA, Scarano L, Cossu E, et al. Percutaneous local ablation of unifocal subclinical breast cancer: clinical experience and preliminary results of cryotherapy. Eur Radiol. 2011;21(11):2344–53.
18. Nurko J, Mabry CD, Whitworth P, Jarowenko D, Oetting L, Potruch T, et al. Interim results from the FibroAdenoma Cryoablation Treatment Registry. Am J Surg. 2005;190(4):647–51; discussion 651–2.
19. Tafra L, Fine R, Whitworth P, Berry M, Woods J, Ekbom G, et al. Prospective randomized study comparing cryo-assisted and needle-wire localization of ultrasound-visible breast tumors. Am J Surg. 2006;192(4):462–70.
20. Jeffrey SS, Birdwell RL, Ikeda DM, Daniel BL, Nowels KW, Dirbas FM, et al. Radiofrequency ablation of breast cancer: first report of an emerging technology. Arch Surg. 1999; 134(10):1064–8.
21. Earashi M, Noguchi M, Motoyoshi A, Fujii H. Radiofrequency ablation therapy for small breast cancer followed by immediate surgical resection or delayed mammotome excision. Breast Cancer. 2007;14(1):39–47.
22. Fornage BD, Sneige N, Ross MI, Mirza AN, Kuerer HM, Edeiken BS, et al. Small (<2-cm) breast cancer treated with US-guided radiofrequency ablation: feasibility study. Radiology. 2004;231(1):215–24.
23. Hayashi AH, Silver SF, van der Westhuizen NG, Donald JC, Parker C, Fraser S, et al. Treatment of invasive breast carcinoma with ultrasound-guided radiofrequency ablation. Am J Surg. 2003;185(5):429–35.
24. Imoto S, Wada N, Sakemura N, Hasebe T, Murata Y. Feasibility study on radiofrequency ablation followed by partial mastectomy for stage I breast cancer patients. Breast. 2009; 18(2):130–4.
25. Manenti G, Bolacchi F, Perretta T, Cossu E, Pistolese CA, Buonomo OC, et al. Small breast cancers: in vivo percutaneous US-guided radiofrequency ablation with dedicated cool-tip radiofrequency system. Radiology. 2009;251(2):339–46.
26. Medina-Franco H, Soto-Germes S, Ulloa-Gómez JL, Romero-Trejo C, Uribe N, Ramirez-Alvarado CA, et al. Radiofrequency ablation of invasive breast carcinomas: a phase II trial. Ann Surg Oncol. 2008;15(6):1689–95.

27. Oura S, Tamaki T, Hirai I, Yoshimasu T, Ohta F, Nakamura R, et al. Radiofrequency ablation therapy in patients with breast cancers two centimeters or less in size. Breast Cancer. 2007;14(1):48–54.
28. Yamamoto N, Fujimoto H, Nakamura R, Arai M, Yoshii A, Kaji S, et al. Pilot study of radiofrequency ablation therapy without surgical excision for T1 breast cancer: evaluation with MRI and vacuum-assisted core needle biopsy and safety management. Breast Cancer. 2011;18(1):3–9.
29. Kinoshita T, Iwamoto E, Tsuda H, Seki K. Radiofrequency ablation as local therapy for early breast carcinomas. Breast Cancer. 2010;18(1):10–7.
30. Fujimoto S, Kobayashi K, Takahashi M, Nemoto K, Yamamoto I, Mutou T, et al. Clinical pilot studies on pre-operative hyperthermic tumour ablation for advanced breast carcinoma using an 8 MHz radiofrequency heating device. Int J Hyperthermia. 2003;19(1):13–22.
31. Marcy P-Y, Magné N, Castadot P, Bailet C, Namer M. Ultrasound-guided percutaneous radiofrequency ablation in elderly breast cancer patients: preliminary institutional experience. Br J Radiol. 2006;80(952):267–73.
32. Susini T, Nori J, Olivieri S, Livi L, Bianchi S, Mangialavori G, et al. Radiofrequency ablation for minimally invasive treatment of breast carcinoma. A pilot study in elderly inoperable patients. Gynecol Oncol. 2007;104(2):304–10.
33. Teh HS, Tan S-M. Radiofrequency ablation – a new approach to percutaneous eradication of benign breast lumps. Breast J. 2010;16(3):334–6.
34. Dooley WC, Vargas HI, Fenn AJ, Tomaselli MB, Harness JK. Focused microwave thermotherapy for preoperative treatment of invasive breast cancer: a review of clinical studies. Ann Surg Oncol. 2010;17(4):1076–93.
35. Gardner RA, Vargas HI, Block JB, Vogel CL, Fenn AJ, Kuehl GV, et al. Focused microwave phased array thermotherapy for primary breast cancer. Ann Surg Oncol. 2002;9(4):326–32.
36. Campbell AM, Land DV. Dielectric properties of female human breast tissue measured in vitro at 3.2 GHz. Phys Med Biol. 1992;37(1):193–210.
37. Vargas HI, Dooley WC, Gardner RA, Gonzalez KD, Venegas R, Heywang-Kobrunner SH, et al. Focused microwave phased array thermotherapy for ablation of early-stage breast cancer: results of thermal dose escalation. Ann Surg Oncol. 2004;11(2):139–46.
38. Vargas HI, Dooley WC, Fenn AJ, Tomaselli MB, Harness JK. Study of preoperative focused microwave phased array thermotherapy in combination with neoadjuvant anthracycline-based chemotherapy for large breast carcinomas. Cancer Therapy. 2007;5(2):401–8.
39. Dooley WC, Vargas HI, Fenn AJ, Tomaselli MB, Harness JK. Randomized study of preoperative focused microwave phased array thermotherapy for early-stage invasive breast cancer. Cancer Therapy. 2008;6(2):395–408.
40. Vargas HI, Dooley WC, Gardner RA, Gonzalez KD, Heywang-Kobrunner SH, Fenn AJ. Success of sentinel lymph node mapping after breast cancer ablation with focused microwave phased array thermotherapy. Am J Surg. 2003;186(4):330–2.
41. Zhou W, Zha X, Liu X, Ding Q, Chen L, Ni Y, et al. US-guided percutaneous microwave coagulation of small breast cancers: a clinical study. Radiology. 2012;263(2):364–73.
42. Trelles MA, Pardo L, Chamorro JJ, Bonanad E, Allones I, Buil C, et al. Erbium:YAG laser as a method of deepithelization in corrective and reductive breast surgery. Ann Plast Surg. 2005;55(2):122–6.
43. Akimov AB, Seregin VE, Rusanov KV, Tyurina EG, Glushko TA, Nevzorov VP, et al. Nd:YAG interstitial laser thermotherapy in the treatment of breast cancer. Lasers Surg Med. 1998;22(5):257–67.
44. Bloom KJ, Dowlat K, Assad L. Pathologic changes after interstitial laser therapy of infiltrating breast carcinoma. Am J Surg. 2001;182(4):384–8.
45. Dowlatshahi K, Francescatti DS, Bloom KJ, Jewell WR, Schwartzberg BS, Singletary SE, et al. Image-guided surgery of small breast cancers. Am J Surg. 2001;182(4):419–25.
46. Haraldsdóttir KH, Ivarsson K, Götberg S, Ingvar C, Stenram U, Tranberg K-G. Interstitial laser thermotherapy (ILT) of breast cancer. Eur J Surg Oncol. 2008;34(7):739–45.

47. Vlastos G, Verkooijen HM. Minimally invasive approaches for diagnosis and treatment of early-stage breast cancer. Oncologist. 2007;12(1):1–10.
48. Bosch MAAJVD, Daniel BL. MR-guided interventions of the breast. Magn Reson Imaging Clin N Am. 2005;13(3):505–17.
49. Mumtaz H, Hall-Craggs MA, Wotherspoon A, Paley M, Buonaccorsi G, Amin Z, et al. Laser therapy for breast cancer: MR imaging and histopathologic correlation. Radiology. 1996;200(3):651–8.
50. Dowlatshahi K, Wadhwani S, Alvarado R, Valadez C, Dieschbourg J. Interstitial laser therapy of breast fibroadenomas with 6 and 8 year follow-up. Breast J. 2010;16(1):73–6.
51. Van Esser S, Stapper G, van Diest PJ, van den Bosch MAAJ, Klaessens JHGM, Mali WPTM, et al. Ultrasound-guided laser-induced thermal therapy for small palpable invasive breast carcinomas: a feasibility study. Ann Surg Oncol. 2009;16(8):2259–63.
52. Harries SA, Amin Z, Smith ME, Lees WR, Cooke J, Cook MG, et al. Interstitial laser photocoagulation as a treatment for breast cancer. Br J Surg. 1994;81(11):1617–9.
53. Novian Health Inc. American Breast Laser Ablation Therapy Evaluation (ABLATE) In: ClinicalTrials.gov [Internet]. 2011. Available from: http://www.clinicaltrials.gov/ct2/show/study/NCT00807924. Cited 7 Apr 2011. p. NLMIdentifier:NCT00807924. http://www.nlm.nih.gov/services/ctcite.html
54. Lynn JG, Zwemer RL, Chick AJ, Miller AE. A new method for the generation and use of focused ultrasound in experimental biology. J Gen Physiol. 1942;26(2):179–93.
55. Chen L, Bouley D, Yuh E, D'Arceuil H, Butts K. Study of focused ultrasound tissue damage using MRI and histology. J Magn Reson Imaging. 1999;10(2):146–53.
56. McDannold N, Hynynen K, Wolf D, Wolf G, Jolesz F. MRI evaluation of thermal ablation of tumors with focused ultrasound. J Magn Reson Imaging. 1998;8(1):91–100.
57. Van Esser S, Veldhuis WB, Van Hillegersberg R, van Diest PJ, Stapper G, ElOuamari M, et al. Accuracy of contrast-enhanced breast ultrasound for pre-operative tumor size assessment in patients diagnosed with invasive ductal carcinoma of the breast. Cancer Imaging. 2007;7:63–8.
58. Furusawa H, Namba K, Nakahara H, Tanaka C, Yasuda Y, Hirabara E, et al. The evolving nonsurgical ablation of breast cancer: MR guided focused ultrasound (MRgFUS). Breast Cancer. 2007;14(1):55–8.
59. Hynynen K, McDannold N, Mulkern RV, Jolesz FA. Temperature monitoring in fat with MRI. Magn Reson Med. 2000;43(6):901–4.
60. Rieke V, Butts Pauly K. Echo combination to reduce proton resonance frequency (PRF) thermometry errors from fat. J Magn Reson Imaging. 2008;27(3):673–7.
61. Hynynen K, Pomeroy O, Smith DN, Huber PE, McDannold NJ, Kettenbach J, et al. MR imaging-guided focused ultrasound surgery of fibroadenomas in the breast: a feasibility study. Radiology. 2001;219(1):176–85.
62. Furusawa H, Namba K, Thomsen S, Akiyama F, Bendet A, Tanaka C, et al. Magnetic resonance-guided focused ultrasound surgery of breast cancer: reliability and effectiveness. J Am Coll Surg. 2006;203(1):54–63.
63. Gianfelice D, Khiat A, Amara M, Belblidia A, Boulanger Y. MR imaging-guided focused US ablation of breast cancer: histopathologic assessment of effectiveness – initial experience. Radiology. 2003;227(3):849–55.
64. Wu F, Wang Z-B, Cao Y-D, Zhu X-Q, Zhu H, Chen W-Z, et al. "Wide local ablation" of localized breast cancer using high intensity focused ultrasound. J Surg Oncol. 2007;96(2):130–6.
65. Huber PE, Jenne JW, Rastert R, Simiantonakis I, Sinn HP, Strittmatter HJ, et al. A new noninvasive approach in breast cancer therapy using magnetic resonance imaging-guided focused ultrasound surgery. Cancer Res. 2001;61(23):8441–7.
66. Wu F, Wang Z-B, Cao Y-D, Chen W-Z, Bai J, Zou J-Z, et al. A randomised clinical trial of high-intensity focused ultrasound ablation for the treatment of patients with localised breast cancer. Br J Cancer. 2003;89(12):2227–33.

67. Gianfelice D, Khiat A, Boulanger Y, Amara M, Belblidia A. Feasibility of magnetic resonance imaging-guided focused ultrasound surgery as an adjunct to tamoxifen therapy in high-risk surgical patients with breast carcinoma. J Vasc Interv Radiol. 2003;14(10):1275–82.
68. Zippel D, Papa M. The use of MR imaging guided focused ultrasound in breast cancer patients; a preliminary phase one study and review. Breast Cancer. 2005;12(1):32–8.
69. Gombos E, Kacher D, Furusawa H, Namba K. Breast focused ultrasound surgery with magnetic resonance guidance. Top Magn Reson Imaging. 2006;17(3):181.
70. Bitton RR, Kaye E, Dirbas FM, Daniel BL, Pauly KB. Toward MR-guided high intensity focused ultrasound for presurgical localization: focused ultrasound lesions in cadaveric breast tissue. J Magn Reson Imaging. 2012;35(5):1089–97.
71. Schmitz AC, van den Bosch MAAJ, Rieke V, Dirbas FM, Butts Pauly K, Mali WPTM, et al. 3.0-T MR-guided focused ultrasound for preoperative localization of nonpalpable breast lesions: an initial experimental ex vivo study. J Magn Reson Imaging. 2009;30(4):884–9.
72. Lopez JK, Bassett LW. Invasive lobular carcinoma of the breast: spectrum of mammographic, US, and MR imaging findings. Radiographics. 2009;29(1):165–76.

Chapter 9
Thoracic Ablation: Primary Lung Cancer, Metastases, Chest Wall Disease

Shuvro Roy-Choudhury

Clinical Features

- Lung tumors are common, accounting for nearly a third of all cancer deaths in the USA.
- Lobar resection or pneumonectomy with mediastinal node sampling/clearance remains the gold standard to achieve a cure in NSCLC, but only 20% of primary lung tumors present with surgically resectable disease and many of these patients are surgically unfit due to comorbidities.
- Lungs are also the second common site for metastasis. Surgical resection for paucimetastatic lung lesions from selected primaries have been proven to offer survival advantage. But repeated resections decrease the amount of functioning lung parenchyma. Metastasis from colon, kidney, breast, sarcoma, and melanoma are particularly suitable. Slow-growing tumors or ones that have a long latent period between primary tumor and metastasis have a better prognosis.
- External beam radiotherapy in surgically unfit cases have a high rate of local recurrence and 15–20% 5-year survival.
- Minimally invasive techniques like radiofrequency, microwave, or cryoablation of primary and secondary lung tumors is a relatively recent minimally invasive modality to treat limited volume lung tumors.
- These newer techniques have mostly been used in a curative setting, although there may be a role to alleviate pain in chest wall disease or to reduce tumor bulk in a palliative setting.
- Although several reports talk about alternative forms of ablation, this chapter will mainly reflect on experience with radiofrequency ablation, the most commonly

S. Roy-Choudhury, FRCS, FRCR, FCIRSE, EBIR
Diagnostic and Interventional Radiology, Fortis Hospitals,
#730, Anandapur EM Bypass Road, Kolkata, West Bengal 700107, India

Consultant Radiologist, Heart of England NHS Foundation Trust, Birmingham, B9 5SS, UK
e-mail: shuvrorc@googlemail.com

T. Clark, T. Sabharwal (eds.), *Interventional Radiology Techniques in Ablation*,
Techniques in Interventional Radiology,
DOI 10.1007/978-0-85729-094-6_9, © Springer-Verlag London 2013

used modality. The principles of radiofrequency, microwave, and cryotherapy have been described elsewhere, but in theory, microwave and cryotherapy offers a number of advantages over radiofrequency in the setting of a solid lesion in an aerated lung parenchyma, particularly when close to large vessels or bronchi.

Diagnostic Evaluation

Clinical

- The patient would have normally be discussed in a multidisciplinary meeting.
- It is preferable to see the patient prior to the procedure and preconsent. This can be nurse-led.
- Patient should have a thorough understanding of the procedure, its rationale, potential complications, and the need for follow up postoperatively.
- Anesthetic review in cases of primary lung tumor – as invariably multiple comorbidities coexist.
- Stop aspirin or clopidogrel 7–15 days prior to the procedure unless absolutely necessary.
- A patient information leaflet is provided.

Laboratory

- Full Blood Count including platelets
- INR
- Respiratory function tests, particularly FEV1. This normally would have been done prior to the lung ablation referral

Imaging

- Staging CT scan: To assess the size, number, location, proximity of important structures, amount of pleural/fissural contact, etc. To assess for extrathoracic disease
- PET: These are usually performed prior to RFA – mainly to assess for nodal or extrathoracic uncontrollable disease
- Pre-operative biopsy

Primary lung tumor: Normally, this would have been performed prior to the lung ablation referral. For patients with poor lung function, this can be a useful marker as to how the patient will cope with the ablation. In exceptional cases, it is reasonable to perform RFA for a suspicious-looking nodule on CT that shows uptake on PET. In my practice, a biopsy is then performed at the time of ablation.

Metastatic lung tumor: Biopsies are usually not necessary. New appearance of a lesion or increase in size of a nodule in a patient with a suitable primary malignancy usually suffice for diagnosis.

Indications

Curative Setting

- Primary non-small-cell lung tumor T1NOMO or small T2NOMO in patients unfit for surgery or does not want surgery
- Best for tumors less than 3 cm. Noncurative for tumors more than 5 cm.
- Lung metastasis from selected slow-growing primaries: Usually, up to 3 per lung and each less than 4 cm. However, more metastasis can be sequentially treated.

Palliative Setting

- May have a role in a cytoreductive/adjuvant setting in stage 3 and 4 lung cancer. Tumor ablation can be combined with radiotherapy, chemotherapy, or chemoembolization, often with synergistic effect.
- Ablation for painful chest wall or bone metastasis offers excellent pain control and reduced analgesia requirement.

Contraindications

- Pneumonectomy. Although ablation postpneumonectomy have been reported, it is best to avoid these patients at the start of practice. Sometimes, the single lung may be functional, i.e., a fibrotic residual lobe post lobectomy may not be able to withstand a transient pneumothorax in the opposite treating side. In this setting, sometimes the staging CT may be misleading. A peek at the CXR is often more useful to assess this.
- FEV1 < 0.8. This is relative, as it is feasible to treat patients with FEV1 between 0.6 and 0.8, provided optimized respiratory and anesthetic support is available.
- Within 1 cm of a large bronchus, blood vessel, or the heart: This is relative – as lesions abutting the pericardium, diaphragm, or large vessels have been treated.

- Pacemakers are usually a contraindication, but ablations have been performed under cardiological supervision.

Patient Preparation

- Admitted in the morning of the procedure
- IV access
- Antibiotic prophylaxis
- Standard GA preparations, including nil orally for 6 h

Relevant Anatomy

Normal Anatomy

- Aerated lung parenchyma around a tumor limits heat conduction, thereby creating an oven effect and keeping the applied heat within the tumor. Conversely, if a tumor has infiltrating margins – this may not treat very well because of the insulating effect of the air. Microwave ablation is theoretically superior to radiofrequency ablation in this regard. With cryoablation, there is progressively improved thermal conductivity as ablation progresses, as pulmonary fluid fills alveolar spaces resulting in reduced times for freeze – thaw cycles. Cryotherapy may also cause less damage to surrounding mediastinal structures or bronchi.
- It is important to understand the lobar anatomy of the lung. Bronchopulmonary segments are not relevant during ablation.
- Location of fissures determines access routes and chances of pneumothorax.
- Mediastinal structures like heart and hilum – usually tumors within 1 cm of these structures are not treated.
- Pulmonary vessels and bronchi – large vessels >3 mm abutting the tumor may cause heat sink, as the pulmonary vessels are subject to 100% of right heart blood flow. Cryotherapy or microwave ablation may be more suitable than radiofrequency in this setting. Equally, uniquely in the lung, a large bronchus may also cause heat sink due to airflow. Moreover, if a large bronchus abuts a peripheral tumor, there is an increased risk of bronchopleural fistula. It is best to monitor such a patient for 2–3 days before discharge.

Aberrant Anatomy

Not usually relevant apart from presence of accessory fissures

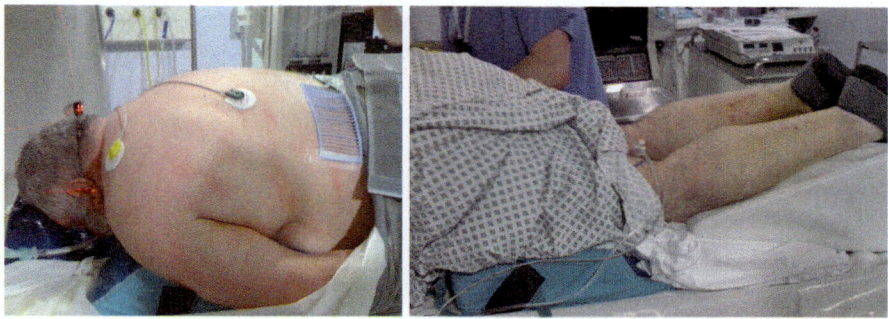

Fig. 9.1 General anesthesia in lung RFA: Close participation with the anesthetic team is required in these patients who invariably have high comorbidities. Pressure points need to be protected, prone GA carries extra risk and long tubings are needed to get in and out of the CT gantry

Equipment

- Standard ablation equipment including generator, electrode, and grounding pad. All electrodes are different and it is useful to get used to one kit. The deficiency of each kit can be made up by increasing user experience. All available electrodes can be used to treat a given lesion; however, clearly, some lesions would be more suited to an individual electrode system. For example, a small metastasis close to the bifurcation of two major arteries is best treated by a needle or solitary electrode while a large target lesion is probably best treated with microwave or a sequential RFA system.
- CT suite: CT fluoroscopy reduces procedure time considerably at the cost of increased radiation exposure to the operator. It is worth spending some time with the technicians to sort out the reconstruction interval and algorithm for each CT acquisition that the operator is comfortable with, to speed up the procedure.
- GA apparatus – Remote anesthesia makes the anesthetists uncomfortable. Prior discussions and an on-site assessment to look at the facilities of the CT suite is useful. The usual anesthetic equipment including Boyle's apparatus, intubation equipment, and drugs are necessary. Peculiar to RFA is the need for a long airway tube to ensure passage within the CT gantry, adequate gel supports to take care of pressure points – particularly in prone position (see Fig. 9.1)
- Standard angiography draping set
- Skin cleanser
- Local anesthetic needle and spinal needle
- Size 11 blade
- Attaching grounding pads (for nonbipolar kits): Depends on the manufacturer. Usually two to four pads are applied – typically in the medial and posterior aspects of both thighs. Hip replacements are not contraindications to RFA – the position of the grounding pads may be altered based on metalwork in the body.
- Suction apparatus

- A pneumothorax kit with an appropriate water seal drainage system. Ideally, a proprietary one-way Heimlich valve, a Seldinger 6–8F drainage kit, and a formal chest drain set should all be present

Preprocedure Medications

- Antibiotic
- Sedation if necessary

Procedure

Planning an Access Route

- Location of a lesion in relation to the intercostal space may change significantly in different phases of breathing.
- The principles of a standard needle biopsy apply: usually, the shortest, straightest route to the lesion avoiding fissures and large blood vessels or bronchi is chosen.
- Subpleural lesions behind a rib are notoriously difficult to get an accurate needle position into and to do overlapping ablations. A scan in a different phase of respiration may be useful. Sometimes, a long straight access from the parenchymal aspect is better.
- The access angle and location often depends on the lesion size, shape, and the corresponding predicted ablation geometry. A thorough understanding of the predicted 3D ablation geometry and a mental coregistration is essential for good planning. This depends on the kit used. For example, a single electrode produces an elliptical ablation volume, a cluster electrode produces a clover-leaf-shaped ablation volume, while the tined electrodes produce more spherical ablation volumes. The LeVeen electrode produces a sphere, which is flatter at the poles, i.e., it produces an ablation that is slightly wider than the axis along the needle. For tined electrodes, typically an entry along the long axis helps – as then – overlapping ablations simply means withdrawing the needle along the same axis rather than a complete new access.
- The access point(s) are then marked with indelible ink.

Positioning the Patient

- It is essential to ensure that the CT table is set to an appropriate height to accomodate the electrode apparatus that sticks out of the patient. This varies from system to system. For example, the table height should be low for obese patients, for noncoaxial or nonflexible systems, and for superficial lesions.

- Prone positioning or the location of the scapula may change access route completely. Position of the arms above the head or alongside the body will also change the scapular position. If in doubt, it is useful to perform a CT in the desired position prior to the GA.
- In prone patients, suitable support to ensure abdominal breathing is required to prevent ventilatory compromise. Other pressure points also need protection.
- If lateral access is contemplated, it is good to ensure that enough space is present between gantry and the patient to accomodate the electrode apparatus outside the body. This can be done by placing the patient off-center on the CT table. This is particularly true if a noncoaxial system is used.

Performing the Procedure

Technique

- Skin preparation: A chlorhexidine or betadine skin preparation is used. A wide area is prepped as a pneumothorax drain may have to be placed at a site remote from the electrode entry site.
- Local anesthesia: This is not required in GA patients. Nevertheless, a 21-G needle with some anesthetic is used to assess needle angle and location prior to the larger electrode. Do not hover at the pleural surface with this needle – it is quite easy to do so with this needle in thin cachectic patients and giving them a pneumothorax prior to start of the procedure !!
- A small skin incision is made
- The electrode is inserted in the desired angle to the appropriate depth. I use a clock face and take the help of an assistant to monitor the angle of entry from the foot end of the CT table. The precise location of the needle tip within the lesion also depends on the electrode and its ablation geometry. The more rounded tines of the LeVeen electrode means that the needle tip should be just beyond the midpoint of the lesion, while the forward pushing tines of the Starburst electrode means that the tip should be short of the midpoint of the lesion.
- If a coaxial needle is used, a biopsy can be performed at this stage through the same needle. A core biopsy can and does cause hemorrhage. So, only perform this, if, it is absolutely necessary.
- Hemorrhage from the biopsy or the needle tract can obscure a lesion very quickly. It is useful to get a quick needle entry into the lesion and commence ablation. This is a good way to stop the bleeding.
- If a pneumothorax occurs during entry, it is usually possible to drain it and complete the ablation.
- The electrode is partially deployed (in case of tined electrodes) and its position checked with a volume CT acquisition. An MPR of this is performed at the

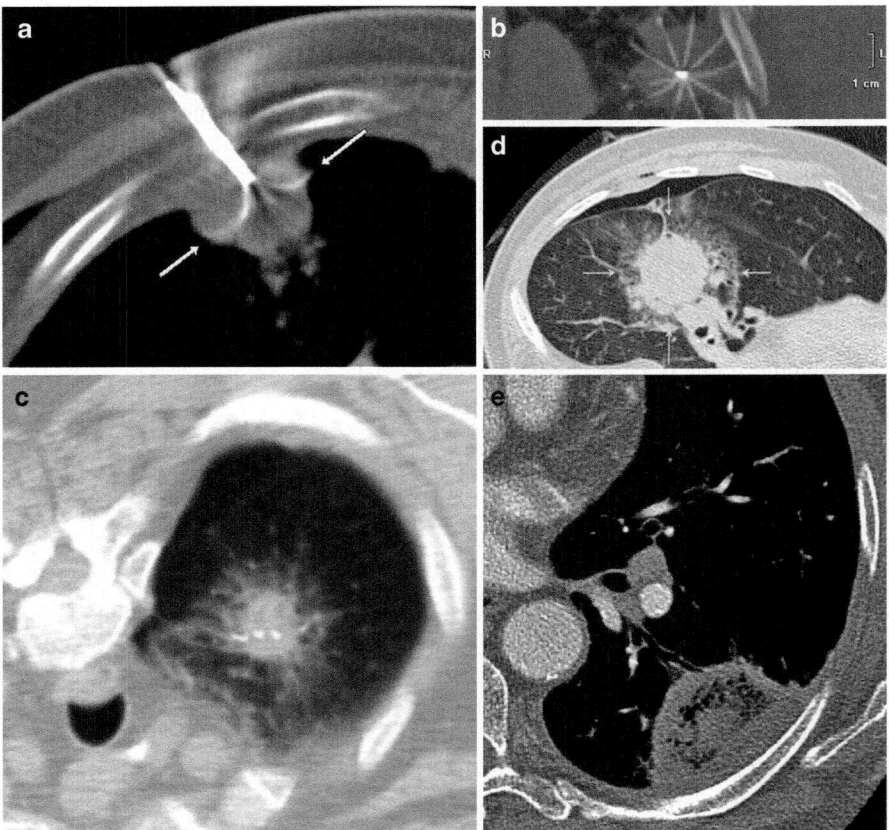

Fig. 9.2 The electrode is partially deployed (in case of tined electrodes) and its position checked with a volume CT acquisition (**a**). An MPR of this is performed at the workstation to ensure that the needle is appropriately centered in all planes before full deployment (**b**). End point of ablation in two different patients (**c** & **d**) with a ground glass opacity all around the tumour. This needs to be checked in all three planes. Sometimes the ablated area appears as bubble lucencies (**e**) that disappear by three months

workstation to ensure that the needle is appropriately centered in all planes before full deployment (see Fig. 9.2). Ideally, tines going through the tumor into normal lung tissue should not be withdrawn, without ablating, for fear of seeding.

- The electrode is fully deployed and its position checked with CT. Once deployed, tined electrode does not move in relation to the lesion.
- Ablation is commenced and continued according to the manufacturer's algorithm. Unlike solid organ ablation, it is necessary to keep a close eye at the needle position, the compliance graph of the Boyle's apparatus, etc. as a pneumothorax may happen mid-procedure and the needle position can change in the lungs.
- A second or subsequent ablation cycles are performed as deemed fit to ensure that there will be an adequate margin all around the tumor.

- The pads can heat up during prolonged ablation. Frequent checks or use of an ice-pack may be useful.
- Track ablation is performed within the lungs, but not across the pleural surface.
- The needle entry site is covered by a small dressing.

Tips

- For lesions close to the pleural surface, or, on the diaphragm, hydrodissection can be used to protect the chest wall or to ensure complete treatment. Algorithms are also different for lesions with pleural contact.
- Often, a significant change in needle angle can be made within the lung without having to withdraw the needle across the pleural surface.
- A small lesion may be enveloped in tines rather than trying to penetrate it by putting the needle tip next to it.
- The 14-G electrodes cause significant flare artefact on CT. Using thicker sections to view or using a bone window can be useful.
- With tined electrodes, angulation of the shaft prior to deployment can change the coverage by the tines considerably.
- With tined electrodes, it is possible to pull the deployed tines away from a vital structure during ablation.
- Hypervascular chest wall lesions and certain parenchymal metastasis can be pre-embolized (intercostal or internal mammary) prior to ablation.
- Pneumothorax may happen at the time of needle withdrawal. A check CT should be performed prior to reversal of the patient.

Endpoint

The endpoint is dictated by the algorithm of the generator when a treatment cycle is completed. Usually, more than one ablation cycle is necessary to encompass the entire tumor with a satisfactory margin. A ground glass halo, around the tumor, measuring at least 5 mm indicates satisfactory endpoint of treatment. (Fig. 9.2) Larger margins are desirable for adenocarcinomas.

Immediate Postprocedure Care

Usual anesthetic recovery principles apply. An additional anesthetic assistant is invaluable for this period, particularly if more than one case is scheduled for the list. Oxygen saturation is monitored continuously, particularly if a pneumothorax had occurred at the time of treatment.

Follow-up and Postprocedure Medications

- A chest radiograph is performed 4 h after the procedure. Good communication with the admitting team is essential.
- A 5-day course of antibiotics is prescribed only in high-risk cases (previous radiotherapy, poor lung function, etc.).
- Patients usually recover very fast and are encouraged to sit up and have a meal in the evening.
- A visit by the operating team on the first post-op day is essential. Pain control, particularly for pleural-based lesions is important. It is important to impress on the clinical team and the admitting nurses that in spite of no apparent scars, etc. the procedure can be painful !!
- Uncomplicated cases may be discharged on the first post-op day with suitable advice regarding postembolization syndrome and pain due to pleural reaction that may be delayed till day 5. Preemptive analgesia is useful. Drained pneumothoraces and lesions close to the pleural surface or those with potential bronchial communication are kept for at least one additional day as delayed pneumothoraces can occur.

Imaging follow-up schedule includes a pre- and postcontrast CT at 1, 4, 7, 12, 18, 24, 36, 48, and 60 months. In cases of renal dysfunction, diffusion-weighted MRI is useful. We use PET as a problem-solving tool, but there is increasing evidence to perform a routine PET at 3–6 months. Interpreting imaging appearances can be complex, but a pattern-based approach can help, as outlined below.

Immediate Postprocedure Appearances on CXR and CT

These include dependent hypostatic changes (normal), a ground glass opacity (GGO) encompassing the tumor, hemorrhage, pleural reactions, etc.

Appearances of Complete Response

- A GGO encompassing the tumor in all planes is the best predictor for complete treatment. This may evolve into an area of atelectasis, the size of which is typically larger than the original tumor at the 1-month scan, which is taken as the baseline for follow-up. The size of the atelectasis reduces over time and eventually becomes a scar. (Fig. 9.3)
- Lack of enhancement between an unenhanced and a postcontrast scan signifies complete necrosis. Ideally, the postcontrast scan should be performed at around 60 s rather than in the arterial phase. (Fig. 9.4)

- Cavitation can be seen in 25% cases and appears between 1 and 4 months.
- Linear strands or bubble lucencies may appear within the treated area (Fig. 9.2).

Appearances of Incomplete Response or Recurrence

Local recurrence is characterized on CT by
- Enlargement of the ablation zone after 1 month,
- Increased enhancement (by at least 15 HU from the unenhanced scan).
- Nodular excrescence from the smooth outline of the treated atelectasis (Fig. 9.5).
- Recurrence can also be due to satellite nodules, needle tract seeding, mediastinal node involvement, further lung nodules, or extrathoracic metastasis.

Results

Detailed literature review is outside the scope of this text, but a summary of the important papers is given in Table 9.1. Complete tumor necrosis and good local control is the goal of ablative therapy. If small tumors are chosen and a good margin of groundglass opacity is obtained at the end of ablation, a local recurrence rate of less than 10% can be achieved, which is similar to the rates achieved by sublobar resection of small lung tumors. Lung function is well preserved after tumor ablation. In a recent paper by Lee H et al., median survival times for patients treated with surgery alone and RFA alone for stage I–II primary lung cancer were 33.8 and 28.2 months, respectively ($p=0.426$). Median survival times for patients treated with chemotherapy alone and RFA with chemotherapy for stage III–IV cancer were 29 and 42 months, respectively ($p=0.03$).

Alternative Therapies

- Surgery: Lobectomy with node sampling is the gold standard for operable and fit Stage 1 and 2 NSCLC, but has higher morbidity and a mortality rate of around 2.5%. Sublobar resections are limited to less fit patients or patients with metastasis. Neoadjuvant therapies may render higher-stage tumors operable.
- External beam radiotherapy: For medically inoperable patients and early stage disease. High local recurrence rate.
- Chemotherapy: For higher-stage disease or used in the neoadjuvant setting.
- Stereotactic radiotherapy: Excellent recent results. May have equivalent survival to lobectomy for small lung cancers with very low morbidity and mortality.
- TACE or arterial infusion therapies: Encouraging results but limited data.

Table 9.1 Literature review

Author (year)	Patients (tumors)	Modality	Pathology	Local recurrence/residual disease (%)	Survival	Complications
deBaère (2006)	60 (100)	RFA	NSCLC Mets	12	71% OS at 12 m	9% treated Ptx
Lencioni (2008)	106 (183)	RFA	NSCLC Mets	12	92%, 70%	25% Ptx, 4% pleural effusion
Hiraki et al. (2007)	128 (342)	RFA	Mets NSCLC	N/A	84%, –, 66%	
Chua et al. (2010)	100	RFA	Colorectal met	N/A	87%, 66%, 50% 30%	23% treated Ptx, 1 emphysema
Hiraki et al. (2011)	50	RFA	NSCLC	31	100%, 93%, 80%	12% grade 2, 6% grade 3 toxicity
Wolf et al. (2008)	50 (82)	MWA		26	83%, 73%, 61%	Ptx (30%), hemoptysis, skin burns
Chan et al. (2011)	19 (23)	CRA	N/A	21.7	N/A	15% Ptx

Survival is cancer specific and at 1,2, 3, and 5 years unless stated

MWA microwave ablation, *RFA* radiofrequency ablation, *CRA* cryoablation, *Ptx* pneumothorax

- Combination treatments: Multimodality combination therapies seems to be the future of lung cancer management.

Complications

Lung is perhaps the riskiest organ to ablate. Prior experience in liver or kidney ablation is useful.

- Pneumothorax is the most common complication (median 28%), occurs more commonly in emphysema and with positive pressure ventilation. It requires drainage/aspiration in around 15% cases. Most pneumothoraces are minor, non-progressive, and do not require any treatment. Rarely, a surgical chest drain is necessary for persistent pneumothorax or a broncho-pleural communication. Almost always, the ablation treatment can be completed with a chest drain in situ. In most cases, it resolves within 24–48 h of chest drainage. Occasionally, it can be delayed, particularly if the GGO is in contact with the pleural surface.
- Infection: Can take the form of pneumonia or lung abscess and is the major cause of mortality following ablation. Previous DXT and age are risk factors.
- Bleeding. Life-threatening in 0.4%. Less severe hemoptysis is seen in around 5%. More with multitined electrode, in basal and mid-zone nodules, with longer needle tracts, and low platelets.
- Postembolization syndrome: Relatively less common following lung ablation. Can be controlled with paracetamol.
- Pleural effusion and aseptic pleuritis: Most common cause for readmission postablation. Puncture numbers and previous chemotherapy are significant risk factors.
- Air embolism, diaphragm injury, brachial plexus or phrenic nerve injury (usually transient), skin burn (usually with microwave), grounding pad burn, tumor seeding, or GA-related ventilatory complications are rare.

In a large Japanese series of 1,000 ablation procedures in 420 patients, four deaths (0.4%) related to RFA procedures was reported, most from interstitial pneumonia. The major complication rate was 9.8%. Frequent major complications were aseptic pleuritis (2.3%), pneumonia (1.8%), lung abscess (1.6%), bleeding requiring blood transfusion (1.6%), pneumothorax requiring pleural sclerosis (1.6%), followed by bronchopleural fistula (0.4%), brachial nerve injury (0.3%), tumor seeding (0.1%), and diaphragm injury (0.1%).

How to Avoid

- Prepare a good team including a dedicated nurse, an anesthetist, and a CT technologist

- Appropriate patient and lesion selection
- Treat one lung at a time
- Keep at risk patient or lesion admitted for longer

Key Points
- Support from and prior discussion with the thoracic multidisciplinary team is critical
- Multiplanar review of the preprocedure CT is essential to plan access and treatment volumes
- GA is useful but not mandatory
- Overtreatment is the key to success – a ground glass margin of 1 cm or greater all around the tumor reduces risk of recurrence. Complete tumor necrosis and good local control is the goal of ablative therapy.
- Rigorous imaging follow-up is critical – CT is usually performed, although PET at 3–6 months could be better.
- Local nodular recurrence, if detected early, can be successfully retreated.
- Complications (most commonly pneumothorax) do occur, more than RFA of other sites.
- Although less used, microwave ablation, cryoablation, or sequential radiofrequency ablation may offer several advantages over standard unipolar radiofrequency ablation in the lungs.

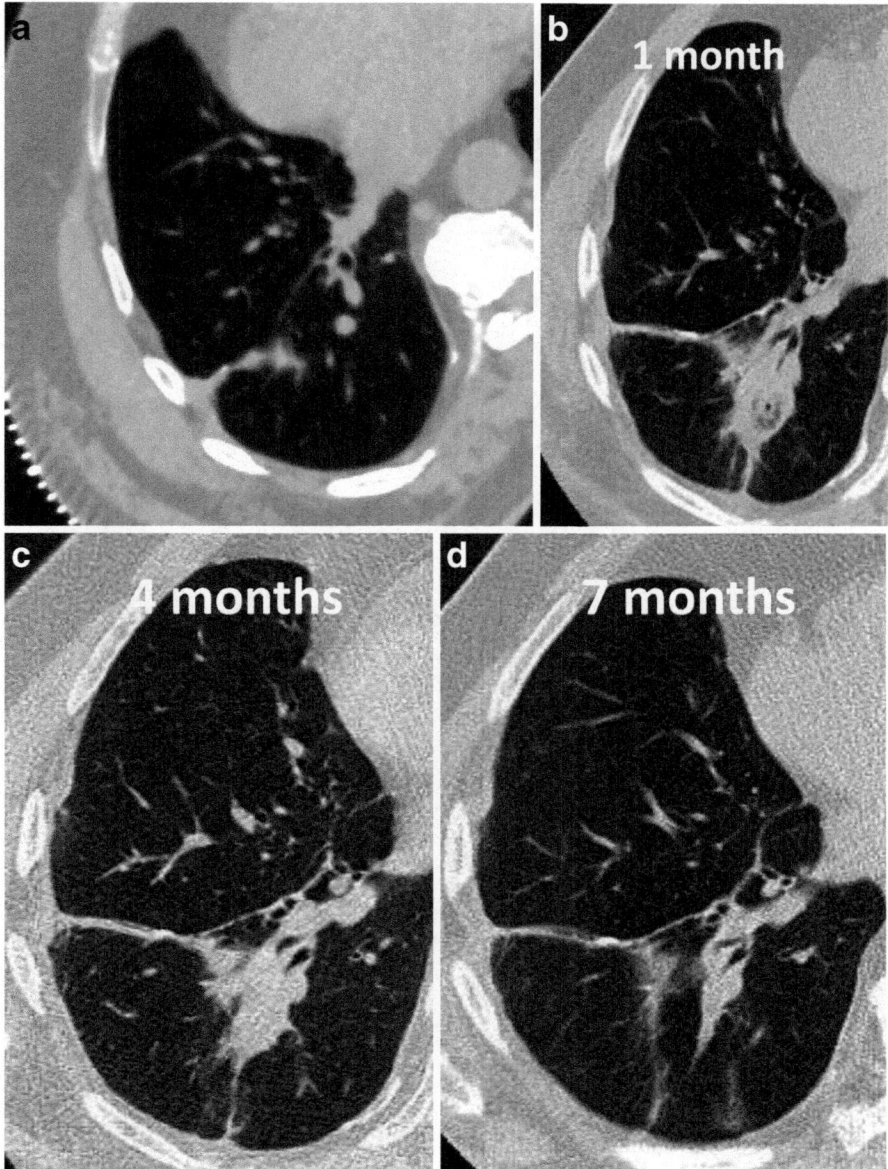

Fig. 9.3 Typical evolution of atelectasis following successful ablation of a small renal cell carcinoma metastasis (**a**). The ablation volume is usually largest at 1 month (**b**) which should be taken as the baseline. From there, the ablation volume should reduce on subsequent follow up (**c**) to eventually become a linear scar (**d**)

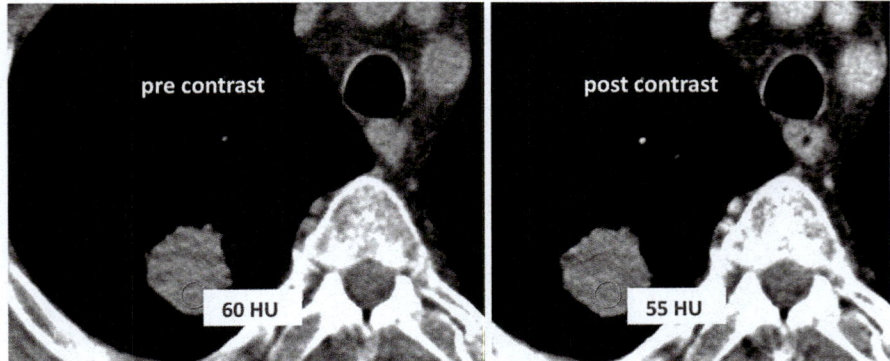

Fig. 9.4 Lack of enhancement of previously enhancing tumours after ablation is a sign of complete treatment

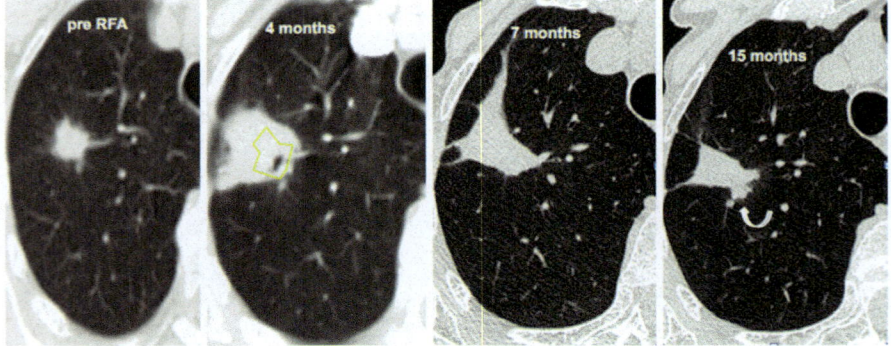

Fig. 9.5 Local recurrence following RFA: Small primary lung tumour treated with RFA. Careful registration of the original lesion on the ablated volume shows absence of adequate margin in the posteromedial aspect of the tumour (**b**). There is a linear atelectasis anteriorly and a small barely perceptible nodule posteriorly at the site of poor margin (**c**). Further follow up at 15 months (**d**) show a clear nodular recurrence where margin was poor, while the atelectasis at the site of adequate margin has disappeared. This was successfully retreated

Suggested Reading

Anderson EM, Lees WR, Gillams AR. Early indicators of treatment success after percutaneous radiofrequency of pulmonary tumors. Cardiovasc Intervent Radiol. 2009;32(3):478–83.

Bojarski JD, Dupuy DE, Mayo-Smith WW. CT imaging findings of pulmonary neoplasms after treatment with radiofrequency ablation: results in 32 tumors. AJR Am J Roentgenol. 2005; 185(2):466–71.

Chan VO, McDermott S, Malone DE, Dodd JD. Percutaneous radiofrequency ablation of lung tumors: evaluation of the literature using evidence-based techniques. J Thorac Imaging. 2011; 26(1):18–26.

de Baère T. Lung tumor radiofrequency ablation: where do we stand? Cardiovasc Intervent Radiol. 2011;34(2):241–51.

de Baère T, Palussière J, Aupérin A, Hakime A, Abdel-Rehim M, Kind M, Dromain C, Ravaud A, Tebboune N, Boige V, Malka D, Lafont C, Ducreux M. Midterm local efficacy and survival after radiofrequency ablation of lung tumors with minimum follow-up of 1 year: prospective evaluation. Radiology. 2006;240(2):587–96.

Deandreis D, Leboulleux S, Dromain C, Auperin A, Coulot J, Lumbroso J, Deschamps F, Rao P, Schlumberger M, de Baère T. Role of FDG PET/CT and chest CT in the follow-up of lung lesions treated with radiofrequency ablation. Radiology. 2011;258(1):270–6.

Fernando HC, Schuchert M, Landreneau R, Daly BT. Approaching the high-risk patient: sublobar resection, stereotactic body radiation therapy, or radiofrequency ablation. Ann Thorac Surg. 2010;89(6):S2123–7.

Kashima M, Yamakado K, Takaki H, Kodama H, Yamada T, Uraki J, Nakatsuka A. Complications after 1000 lung radiofrequency ablation sessions in 420 patients: a single center's experiences. AJR Am J Roentgenol. 2011;197(4):W576–80.

Lee H, Jin GY, Han YM, Chung GH, Lee YC, Kwon KS, Lynch D. Comparison of survival rate in primary non-small-cell lung cancer among elderly patients treated with radiofrequency ablation, surgery, or chemotherapy. Cardiovasc Intervent Radiol. 2012;35(2):343–50.

Lencioni R, Crocetti L, Cioni R, Suh R, Glenn D, Regge D, Helmberger T, Gillams AR, Frilling A, Ambrogi M, Bartolozzi C, Mussi A. Response to radiofrequency ablation of pulmonary tumours: a prospective, intention-to-treat, multicentre clinical trial (the RAPTURE study). Lancet Oncol. 2008;9(7):621–8.

Sonntag PD, Hinshaw JL, Lubner MG, Brace CL, Lee FT Jr. Thermal ablation of lung tumors. Surg Oncol Clin N Am. 2011;20(2):369–87, ix.

Chapter 10
Hepatic Ablation: Hepatocellular Carcinoma and Metastases

Ronald S. Winokur and Daniel B. Brown

Clinical Features

- Hepatocellular carcinoma is the fifth most common cause of cancer in the world and its incidence is increasing worldwide because of the dissemination of Hepatitis B and C infection [1–6].
- Approximately 5–15% of cirrhotic patients with hepatocellular carcinoma meet the criteria for surgical resection [5, 7–11].
- Patients with cirrhosis are at the highest risk of developing hepatocellular carcinoma and should be monitored with imaging every 6 months [12].
- The mortality of patients with hepatocellular carcinoma that is not treated is essentially 100%.
- The liver is the primary and solitary site of metastatic disease in many malignancies including colorectal cancer, neuroendocrine malignancies, and ocular melanoma with approximately 50,000 cases of hepatic metastases from 145,000 new cases of colorectal cancer diagnosed each year [13, 14].
- Unfortunately, because most hepatic metastases are in unresectable locations or in patients with poor hepatic reserve, curative resection is only possible in 20% of patients at the time of presentation in the case of metastatic colorectal carcinoma [15–19].

R.S. Winokur, M.D. • D.B. Brown, M.D. (✉)
Division of Interventional Radiology, Department of Radiology, Thomas Jefferson University Hospital, 132 South 10th Street Suite 766 Main Building, Philadelphia, PA 19003, USA
e-mail: ronald.winokur@jeffersonhospital.org; daniel.brown@jefferson.edu

T. Clark, T. Sabharwal (eds.), *Interventional Radiology Techniques in Ablation*,
Techniques in Interventional Radiology,
DOI 10.1007/978-0-85729-094-6_10, © Springer-Verlag London 2013

Diagnostic Evaluation

Clinical

- During the consent process, be sure to explain to the patient the goals of treatment and present realistic outcomes.
- A preprocedure sedation/anesthesia evaluation should be performed.
- Although ablation can be performed under moderate sedation, thermal ablation with RF ablation or microwave can be painful and the option to undergo general anesthesia should be provided. General anesthesia is also recommended for longer procedures or when targeting will require precise breath holding.

Laboratory

- The following laboratory values should be checked prior to any intervention
  - Complete Blood Count to check hemoglobin/hematocrit, platelet count, and WBC
  - Coagulation Tests including PT, PTT and INR
  - Liver function tests
  - Tumor markers may be checked prior to the procedure in order to obtain a baseline for follow-up

Imaging

- Hepatocellular carcinoma is staged and evaluated with dynamic contrast-enhanced liver MRI and/or a triple-phase CT scan of the liver. CT scan of the chest is also frequently performed, as the lungs are a common metastatic site.
- Patients with metastatic tumors are worked up with CT scan of the chest/abdomen/pelvis and/or a PET CT scan.
- Ultrasound is frequently used as a screening modality for patients with cirrhosis to evaluate for the first mass lesion of HCC, although screening with MRI is becoming more common.

Indications

- Inoperable primary liver tumor due to size/location or poor surgical candidacy from other comorbid diseases.

- Either a single or multicentric HCC with up to three tumors, each preferably less than 3 cm in patients who are not candidates for resection or transplantation [20–22].
- Child-Pugh class A and B for patients with cirrhosis.
- Up to three hepatic metastases less than or equal to 3 cm in a patient that is not an operative candidate.
- East Coast Oncology Group (ECOG) performance status of 0–1.

Contraindications

- Relative Contraindications

  - Close proximity to major vessels due to the "heat sink" effect [23–26]
  - Lesions greater than 5 cm [22, 27]
  - Greater than five hepatic lesions [20]

- Absolute Contraindications

  - Significant extrahepatic disease
  - Child-Pugh class C cirrhosis
  - Active infection
  - Masses that cannot be accessed percutaneously
  - Tumors that occupy greater than 30% of the liver volume [21]
  - Close proximity (1–2 cm) to the central lobar and common bile ducts [21]

Patient Preparation

- The patient should remain NPO (nothing by mouth) for 6 h prior to the procedure. The patient may ingest medications with sips of water in the morning of the procedure.
- Informed consent should be obtained from the patient or an appropriate representative explaining the goals of the procedure and potential immediate complications. The patient should understand the alternatives to undergoing the therapy.
- Warfarin (Coumadin) should be held for 72 h prior to the procedure with coagulation parameters rechecked. If necessary, coagulopathy should be corrected with a target INR of 1.5 or less.
- The platelet count should be 50,000 or more for thermal ablation with planned tract cauterization.
- Aspirin and clopidogrel (Plavix) should be held 5–7 days prior to the procedure to avoid bleeding complications, provided they are not being taken due to drug-eluting coronary stents or other clinical scenario at high risk for interruption of antiplatelet therapy.

Relevant Anatomy

Normal Anatomy

- The liver is the largest abdominal organ occupying the right upper quadrant of the abdomen.
- The stomach, duodenum, and transverse colon border the liver medially. The hepatic flexure of the colon is inferior to the liver. The right kidney and adrenal gland are posterior to the liver.
- The liver has a unique dual blood supply receiving 75% from the portal vein and 25% from the hepatic artery.
- The porta hepatis is a transverse slit in the hilum of the liver that is perforated by the right and left hepatic ducts, hepatic artery, and portal vein.
- The main portal vein divides into the right and left portal veins at the porta hepatis. The right portal vein courses horizontally and bifurcates into anterior and posterior divisions. The left portal vein courses horizontally and turns cranially before dividing into ascending and descending branches.
- The proper hepatic artery is situated anterior to the main portal vein and medial to the common bile duct at the hilum of the liver.
- The proper hepatic artery typically divides into the right, left, and (sometimes) the middle hepatic arteries. The middle hepatic artery, if present, supplies the medial segment of the left hepatic lobe, augmented by branches of the left hepatic artery. Branches of the right hepatic artery typically supply the caudate lobe. The right hepatic artery also gives off the cystic artery.
- The liver can be divided into the right, left, and caudate lobes.

    - The interlobar fissure separating the right and left lobes of the liver consists of the imaginary line drawn between the gallbladder fossa and the middle hepatic vein.
    - The left hepatic lobe is divided into medial and lateral segments by the fissure for the ligamentum teres.
    - The fissure for the ligamentum venosum separates the left hepatic lobe from the caudate lobe.

- The Bismuth-Couinaud system is the most common segmental nomenclature system used.

    - This system divides the liver into eight segments. Segment 1 is the caudate lobe. Segments 2 and 3 represent the superior and inferior lateral segments of the left hepatic lobe. Segment 4 represents the medial segment of the left hepatic lobe and is divided into segment 4a and 4b, which are above and below the level of the left portal vein, respectively. The right hepatic lobe is separated into anterior and posterior by the right hepatic vein and separated into superior and inferior by the right portal vein. The anteroinferior segment is 5, the posteroinferior segment is 6, the posterosuperior segment is 7, and anterosuperior segment is 8.

Anatomic Variants

- Variant anatomy is common in the hepatic vasculature. This anatomy rarely affects planning for ablation procedures.
- The classic arrangement of hepatic arterial anatomy is only seen in 55% of patients. Common variants include an accessory or completely aberrant right hepatic artery arising from the superior mesenteric artery, a partially or completely aberrant left hepatic artery arising from the left gastric artery, and a left hepatic artery giving rise to a middle hepatic artery.
- Anatomic variation in the portal vein can include absence of the right portal vein with anomalous branches from the main portal vein and left portal vein.
- Duplication of, absence of, and accessory hepatic veins can also occur.

Equipment

Percutaneous Ethanol Injection (PEI)

- 95% ethanol used for cases with different injection techniques.
  - 20–22 gauge conical tip needle with multiple side holes with ethanol injected via a syringe and connecting tubing.
  - The Quadra-fuse needle (Rex Medical, Conshohocken, PA) is an expandable needle that allows dispersal of absolute ethanol over a greater area than a standard needle.

Radiofrequency Ablation (RFA)

- Please see Chap. 2 for a complete description of RFA devices.

Microwave Ablation

- Please see Chap. 4 for a complete description of microwave devices.

Cryoablation

- Please see Chap. 3 for a complete description of cryoablation devices.

Preprocedure Medications

- Once the patient is adequately sedated for the procedure, 1% lidocaine is used for local anesthesia at the site of expected probe insertion.
- Preprocedure antibiotics are not universally required and routine use is controversial. Some studies have shown no difference in the development of postprocedure hepatic abscess [28]. However, patients with colonized bile ducts are at increased risk for developing abscesses. These patients have typically had procedures violating the Sphincter of Oddi such as bilioenteric anastomosis, endoscopic sphincterotomy, and either endoscopic or percutaneous stent placement. Patients with diabetes mellitus may be at increased risk for postablation abscess formation as well. In these groups, prophylactic antibiotics covering gram-negative bowel flora are commonly used.

Procedure

Planning an Access Route

- Utilizing the preprocedure imaging (CT, MRI, and/or Ultrasound), a route of entry into the tumor is planned that minimizes the risk of damaging adjacent structures.
- Ablation probes can be inserted under sonographic, CT, or MR guidance using a percutaneous approach.
- Ultrasound is the most commonly used method, but care should be taken to assure that the lesion can be visualized by ultrasound. Even if ultrasound is used to place the electrode, monitoring the ablation with CT may be useful to get a better assessment of adjacent structures.
- If a margin of at least 1 cm cannot be obtained between the active tip within a lesion and a nontarget adjacent structure, adjunctive use of dextrose solution, carbon dioxide, or balloon interposition can be used to separate vital organs [26, 29–31].

Performing the Procedure

- Percutaneous Ethanol Ablation

    – Predominantly performed with ultrasound guidance under conscious sedation. Ethanol induces coagulation necrosis by cellular dehydration, protein denaturation, and chemical occlusion of small tumor vessels [32].

- With multisidehole or endhole needles, a 20–22 gauge needle is inserted into a tumor and small aliquots of 95% ethanol are infused as the needles are withdrawn until the entire tumor is covered as represented by the development of increased echogenicity by ultrasound. Once the tumor is completely echogenic, the needle is left in situ for 5–10 min and withdrawn while aspirating to prevent intraperitoneal spillage. This can be performed as multiple sessions where 1–8 mL of ethanol is injected per session or as a single session technique [33, 34].
- With the Quadra-fuse needle, a 20 and 5 mL syringe are connected via a 3-way stopcock and used to infuse the sideport. One milliliter aliquots are injected with the needle expanded to 1 cm. The tines are retracted and the needle rotated until a 360° circumference is achieved. Following this, the needle is expanded to 2 cm and this process is repeated until either maximal diameter is obtained or the needle is fully expanded [35].

- Radiofrequency Ablation

  - Percutaneous RFA is performed under either conscious sedation or general anesthesia if procedural pain is expected to be problematic or procedure time will be longer than average.
  - The RFA electrode is inserted under image guidance using ultrasound, CT, or MRI.
  - The choice of device, image guidance, and approach is physician-, institution-, and potentially tumor-dependent.
  - Grounding pads are applied to the patient's thighs.
  - The ablation needle is inserted directly into the target tissue and electrodes expanded if appropriate as per the device. Imaging confirming appropriate positioning is obtained. The generator is turned on and a target temperature or impedance is set.
  - Heating of tissue to 50–55°C for 4–6 min produces irreversible cell damage. At temperatures of 60–100°C, near immediate tissue coagulation is produced as a result of irreversible damage to mitochondria and cytosolic enzymes of the cells. At temperatures greater than 100°C, tissue vaporizes and carbonizes [36].
  - The target temperature for RF ablation is 55–100°C.
  - Based on surgery literature, an adequate tumor-free margin of preferably 2 cm and no less than 1 cm is necessary to prevent local progression [16, 22].
  - The heat at a particular distance from the probe dissipates at 1/day where d equals the distance from the probe tip [21, 37].
  - The tumor/surrounding liver environment of an HCC arising within a cirrhotic liver is favorable compared to metastatic disease. This is due to the insulating effect of the cirrhotic liver described as the "oven effect," which allows for higher temperatures to be reached and maintained [38].
  - Most RFA devices produce a maximal ablation zone of 3 cm in diameter. In order to treat tumors larger than 2 cm, overlapping treatments or use of

multiple ablation probes are required to create a larger ablation zone and maintain a 1 cm margin of normal tissue [22].

- The Angiodynamics device reaches its endpoint based on time at temperature and contains thermocouples at the tips of the electrodes, which monitor the tissue temperature.
- The Radiotherapeutics system reaches its endpoint based on elevated tissue impedance. The ablation is performed in a two-step delivery. After impedance reaches 300 Ω, the generator is stopped for 30 s and restarted at a lower energy until impedance "roll-off" recurs.
- The Cool Tip system uses a pulsed delivery system and halts energy delivery for 15 s if tissue impedance rises to 30 Ω greater than baseline. Hepatic ablations are performed for 12 min if a single or cluster electrode is used. For the Switchbox with three separate active electrodes, a 16-min ablation is performed. Final endpoint determination is based on temperature with the cooling pump turned off.
- All systems deliver current via the active portions of the electrodes. Heat is generated by friction from electrical energy resulting in rapidly vibrating cells.
- Ultrasound can be used as a rough guide to monitor the treatment process for increased echogenicity that results from coagulative necrosis of the tissue.

- Microwave Ablation

  - Percutaneous microwave ablation is performed under either conscious sedation or general anesthesia if procedural pain is expected to be problematic or procedure time will be longer than average.
  - As with RFA, local anesthesia is typically obtained with 1% lidocaine. The insertion of microwave ablation probes is typically performed under image guidance with US or CT.
  - The device does not need to be grounded, so grounding pads are not applied as with RFA.
  - Intratumoral temperatures can be measured with a second thermocouple probe.
  - One major difference between RFA and MW ablation is that microwave generates higher temperatures and is less susceptible to heat sink effects.
  - Lethal temperatures to produce coagulation necrosis are similar to RFA.
  - MW ablation can result in a larger zone of active heating due to the broader power density surrounding the microwave antenna [29, 39].
  - When using multiple MW applicators, appropriate spacing must be maintained. If applicators are either too close in proximity or too far apart, the results can be suboptimal.
  - Microwave ablation is also not limited by tissue charring because of its electromagnetic nature resulting in higher temperatures in a shorter period of time.

Immediate Postprocedure Care

* Pain following the procedure is typically not severe unless the ablation included the diaphragm or intercostal/abdominal muscles, or if a subcapsular hematoma formed at the access site. Discomfort can usually be managed with oral analgesics.
* The patient can start on clear liquids in recovery with diet advanced as tolerated.
* The patient typically is discharged from the hospital on the day of the procedure.
* Instructions should be given to contact the IR service if the patient has intractable pain uncontrolled by analgesia or other symptoms.
* The use of postprocedure antibiotics is appropriate for the high-risk patient groups described above.

Follow-up and Postprocedure Medications

* Follow-up after ablation is mainly directed at identifying residual or recurrent tumor within the liver.
* Imaging following the procedure should follow the same protocol used prior to ablation. Multiphase CT and dynamic contrast-enhanced MRI are best able to assess for residual tumor burden. MRI may have slightly higher sensitivity for early local progression compared to CT [40]. If the tumor was hypermetabolic prior to the procedure, PET/CT can also be used to determine tumor viability.
* The first postprocedure imaging study is usually performed at 1 month. If there is not evidence of residual disease at that point, subsequent imaging can be performed at 3-month intervals [22, 40].
* On CT, the ablation cavity is low attenuation without enhancement or solid nodules [22, 41–44]. In the immediate postprocedure period, a hypervascular area may be seen surrounding the ablation zone, which represents increased arterial perfusion and possible inflammatory reaction [42, 44].
* On MRI, the ablated tissue is homogeneously hypointense on T1- and T2-weighted images with hyperintense T2 signal or nodular enhancement concerning residual or recurrent disease [22, 40, 45–47].
* 18-fluorodeoxyglucose (18-FDG)-labeled PET scanning has also been studied to evaluate for tumor recurrence and shows sensitivity for incomplete ablation or tumor recurrence [48–50].
* In addition to imaging, follow-up with tumor markers such as alpha-fetoprotein and CEA is recommended.

Results

Hepatocellular Carcinoma

- The outcome after ablation of hepatocellular carcinoma is highly dependent on tumor size and the presence of underlying cirrhosis.
- Transplantation results in a 5-year survival rate of 70–83% [51].
- Surgical resection results in a 5-year survival rate of 40–70% [25, 52, 53].
- Percutaneous Ethanol Injection (PEI)

  - Percutaneous ethanol injection results in complete necrosis of approximately 70% of small lesions [54].
  - The 5-year survival rates following PEI in patients with Childs A cirrhosis is 41–60% [54–58].
  - The major limitation of PEI is a high local progression rate of 33% in lesions smaller than 3 cm and 43% in larger lesions [59, 60]. The ethanol distributes unevenly within the tumor and it is unable to penetrate intratumoral septations or affect satellite nodules. As HCC increases in size, satellite nodules become larger and more distant from the primary mass.

- Radiofrequency Ablation (RFA)

  - RFA produces complete necrosis of tumors smaller than 3 cm in 80–90% of cases by pathological evaluation and postprocedural imaging showing avascularity [22, 25, 27]. Complete tumor necrosis has been described in 88% of tumors in a nonperivascular location [25]. Outcomes are less impressive in larger masses. Tumors 3.5–5 cm in size are completely necrotic at posttreatment imaging in 50–70% of cases while larger tumors are completely necrotic in less than 50% of cases [27].
  - The 1-, 2-, 3-, 4-, and 5-year survival rates after RF ablation for HCC smaller than 5 cm are 82–97%, 75–86%, 54–77%, 66–68%, and 33–54%, respectively [27, 56, 61–70].
  - The relative value of RF ablation versus resection for HCC is subject to debate. Chen et al. [63] showed no significant difference in overall survival for patients treated with RF ablation and surgical resection for tumors up to 5 cm in size. A recent study by Huang et al. [66] contradicted the findings of Chen et al. [63] showing statistically significant survival benefit for patients undergoing surgical resection compared to RFA. Prospective randomized data do not exist.
  - Three studies comparing PEI to RFA for HCC showed a significant survival benefit at 3 years for patients treated with RFA (3-year survival rate of 74–80%). The corresponding 3-year survival rates following PEI were 50–63% [71–75]. However, two other studies showed no significant difference in 3-year survival between PEI and RFA [76, 77].

- There is also a survival benefit in patients that are naïve to treatment or have less severe underlying cirrhosis. The better outcomes in patients with lesser degrees of liver failure demonstrate the complexity of estimated survival in patients with both cirrhosis and cancer.

  Five-year survival for patients with Childs A cirrhosis is 43–64%, while Childs B cirrhosis patients have 5-year survival of 31–38% [62, 65, 67, 70].

- Microwave Ablation (MWA)

  - Most existing data on MWA is with systems not available in the United States.
  - The 1-, 2-, and 5-year reported survival rates after MWA are 92–96%, 81–83%, and 56%, respectively [78–80].
  - The local progression rate after MWA for HCC is 6–8% [78, 79, 81], which compares favorably to studies of RFA.
  - One study showed no significant difference between RFA and MWA for treatment of HCC, but there was a tendency favoring RFA on the basis of local progression and complication rates [82].

- Cryoablation

  - Only one large cohort study of cryoablation has been performed. This study compared cryoablation plus chemoembolization with cryoablation alone. The study had a large proportion of patients with Child class B cirrhosis and multifocal HCC. The local progression rate was 24% and the 5-year survival rate was 23%. The complication rate of 31% was much higher than that seen with other ablative techniques [83].
  - A smaller study of 36 matched patients compared cryoablation to RFA in patients with HCC smaller than 5 cm. Initial local control was similar among the two groups: 80% for cryoablation and 86% for RFA. The local progression rate was higher for cryoablation (38% versus 17%), but the 1-year survival rate was similar between the two groups: 66% for cryoablation and 61% for RFA [84].

Metastatic Disease

- Colorectal Metastases

  - The second most common use of hepatic ablation after treatment of HCC is in management of colorectal carcinoma metastases.
  - Local control of the tumor was obtained in 78% of patients with tumors smaller than 2.5 cm treated with RFA [83].

- The 1-, 2-, and 3-year survival after treatment with RFA in one study was 93%, 69%, and 46%, respectively [85].
- The 1-, 3-, and 5-year survival from the time of ablation in another study was 97%, 84%, and 40%, respectively. The median survival duration in that study was 59 months [86]. Patients included in this study had tumors smaller than 4 cm.
- Patient outcome and survival in metastatic colorectal carcinoma is highly dependent on the number and size of hepatic metastases as well as extrahepatic disease burden [87].
- The local progression rate after RFA is 18–55% [85, 86, 88–90]. When broken down by tumor size, a recurrence rate of 21.6% was seen for lesions smaller than 2.5 cm and 52.8% for tumors 2.6–4 cm [85].

- Other Hepatic Metastases

  - Limited reports exist in the literature describing the outcomes of patients with metastases from breast cancer or sarcomas to the liver following RFA.
  - Although the use of ablative techniques for inoperable hepatic metastases from various tumors can be estimated from the experience with colorectal cancer, the current literature does not support or refute its use [91].
  - In addition to using ablative therapy for local tumor control, it has been utilized for palliative techniques related to rapidly growing surface tumors and hormonal symptoms from neuroendocrine tumors [92–96].

- No large cohort studies of microwave ablation or cryoablation for hepatic metastases have been performed in the United States. However, the findings seen in hepatocellular carcinoma would theoretically also apply to the management of unresectable metastatic lesions.

Alternative Therapies

- Hepatic transplantation is considered to be the only truly curative treatment for patients with HCC and cirrhosis. However, it is also not a viable treatment for patients with advanced HCC. Transplantation is currently restricted by the Milan Criteria: the patient must have a single tumor less than 5 cm or up to three tumors each less than 3 cm to qualify for transplantation [97, 98]. While other less-restrictive criteria have been proposed, overall tumor burden needs to be limited to be considered for transplantation [99]. The shortage of donor organs also greatly limits the utilization of transplantation.
- Surgical resection of patients with HCC and compensated cirrhosis improves survival with 5-year survival rates of approximately 50–83% [9, 100, 101]. However, surgical resection is associated with significant postoperative morbid-

ity and prolonged recovery. In addition, many patients are not surgical candidates due to tumor location, advanced cirrhosis with insufficient hepatic reserve, or comorbid disease.

- The development of cytostatic targeted therapies is changing the management of patients with HCC [102, 103]. However, the exact role and timing of these therapies is evolving. The initial randomized trial compared sorafenib to supportive care and found a median overall survival of 10.7 and 7.9 months in the treatment and control groups, respectively [103]. Time to progression was 5.5 months in the treatment and 2.8 months in the control groups. A recent study published outcomes when sorafenib was combined with doxorubicin (the previous systemic gold standard therapy for HCC) compared to sorafenib monotherapy [102]. The combination of sorafenib and doxorubicin led to a median survival of 13.7 months versus 6.5 months with sorafenib.
- Endovascular treatment such as transarterial chemoembolization (TACE) radioembolization with Yttrium-90 microspheres is another possibility for patients with both HCC and metastatic disease to the liver if ablative techniques are not possible [104–108].

Complications

- Complications are generally stratified based on the guidelines from the Society of Interventional Radiology (SIR). Major complications result in admission to the hospital for therapy (in outpatients), an unplanned increase in the level of care, prolonged hospitalization, permanent adverse sequelae, or death. Minor complications result in no sequelae, although they may require nominal therapy or a short hospital stay for observation [20].
- Major complications following hepatic RF ablation include intraperitoneal bleeding requiring transfusion, liver abscess, intestinal perforation, pneumothorax and hemothorax, bile duct injury, and seeding of the tract by tumor [20].
- The overall incidence of clinically relevant, major complications including death is approximately 0.9–5.7% [30, 109–111].
- The majority of studies report a mortality rate of much less than 1%, ranging from 0.1% to 0.5% [110, 111]. However, one study with a cohort of 582 patients reported deaths in 1.4% of patients, which may be due to the inhomogeneity of the patient population as both intraoperative and percutaneous therapies were included [28].
- The most common major complication in a study of 2,320 patients and 3,554 lesions was intraperitoneal hemorrhage requiring therapy, which occurred in 12 patients (0.5%) [111]. Seven of the 12 patients had an INR between 1.4 and 1.8. Other studies reported a similar proportion of intraperitoneal hemorrhage requiring transfusion of 0.3–0.5% [28, 109].
- The rate of hepatic abscess after percutaneous hepatic RFA is 0.3% [110, 111].

- Two important risk factors for abscess formation include bacterial colonization of the biliary tract and diabetes mellitus. Bacterial colonization of the biliary system can occur from prior bilioenteric anastomosis, endoscopic sphinctero-tomy, endoscopic or percutaneous stent placement, and bilioenteric fistula.
- Since gas is frequently seen within an ablated lesion on CT, the diagnosis of hepatic abscess should be based on both imaging findings and clinical symptoms [109].
- The treatment of hepatic abscesses should consist of intravenous antibiotics and possibly percutaneous drainage.

- Damage to extrahepatic structures such as the bowel occurs in 0.2–0.3% of patients [28, 111].

  - In the study by Livraghi et al. [111], six out of the seven patients with gastro-intestinal perforation had a history of prior colon resection that resulted in adhesions in the right upper quadrant affixing the bowel to the liver.
  - The colon is considered to be at greater risk for damage and perforation in comparison to the stomach and small bowel due to its lack of mobility and thinner wall [111].
  - Management of damage to the GI tract includes bowel rest, antibiotics, drainage if there is abscess formation, and surgical closure of the enterotomy [109].

- Hemothorax requiring drainage occurs in less than 0.1% of patients [28, 111]. Pneumothorax occurred in 1 out of 2,320 patients in the study by Livraghi et al. [111].

  - The development of pneumothorax and hemothorax is related to use of an intercostal approach to treat masses near the diaphragm or dome of the liver.
  - Since the clinical symptoms of dyspnea cannot be differentiated from pulmo-nary embolism, the appropriate imaging workup of these patients should be performed with an initial chest radiograph followed by a chest CT if the radio-graph does not explain the symptoms [28, 109, 111].

- Biloma caused by thermal ablation has been reported to occur in 0.05–8% of cases [111–115].

  - The majority of bilomas developed within 6 months following treatment and 50% of cases resolved spontaneously without treatment or major complica-tion [116].
  - If patients develop signs of infection, antibiotics and percutaneous drainage may be considered [109].

- The incidence of tumor seeding along the ablation tract is rare with a rate of 0.3–0.5% [28, 111, 117].

  - This complication is exceedingly more common for treatment of HCC com-pared to liver metastases, particularly if a subcapsular tumor is directly punc-tured [118].

- The number of punctures should be minimized, the electrode should be placed so that it traverses a sufficient cuff of normal liver, and cauterization of the electrode tract (i.e. "hot withdrawal") should be performed to minimize the risk of tract seeding [111, 115, 119].
- One group of investigators described a 2.7% tract seeding rate while using an expandable electrode, but these investigators did not perform tract coagulation on withdrawal [119].

- Minor complications or side effects include periprocedural pain, fever, asymptomatic pleural effusion, and grounding pad burns with an overall rate of minor complications ranging from 1.7% to 6.3% [28, 109, 111].
- The postablation syndrome consisting of fever, nausea, vomiting, and right upper quadrant pain is considered a side effect rather than a complication due to its frequency-following treatment.

  - The postablation syndrome results from the release of mediators and inflammatory cytokines. The frequency, severity, and time to onset of the symptoms are directly related to the volume of tissue that is ablated [22, 111].
  - The treatment for the postablation syndrome is supportive with antipyretics and hydration. The condition is self-limiting and can persist up to 2–3 weeks [22].
  - The most important distinction from the postablation syndrome is abscess formation or septicemia. Further investigation with blood cultures and imaging is warranted if there is clinical concern for abscess or sepsis.

- Ablation immediately adjacent to the gallbladder fossa is feasible and results in transient mild ablation induced cholecystitis that is self-limiting and typically resolves without treatment [20, 120]. Perforation of the gallbladder by the RFA probe results in more serious complications, which may require endoscopic or percutaneous drainage [120].
- Pleural effusions are commonly seen with an intercostal approach for tumors at the dome of the liver. The effusions are typically asymptomatic and resolve within 1–2 weeks without therapy [111].
- Skin burns at the site of the grounding pads are infrequently seen complications with a reported rate of 0.2% by the large multicenter trial by Livraghi et al. [111]. They reported this complication in the early phase of technology development when a single grounding pad was used rather than the current standard of multiple grounding pads. The single center study by de Baere et al. [28] with 312 patients reported grounding pad burns in 1.6% of patients.
- PEI is usually well tolerated with an overall rate of major and minor complications of 3.2% in a large multicenter trial [121]. Tract seeding occurred in 0.7% of patients following PEI. Larger volume injections during a single session can result in a higher complication rate [121]. Single session ablation is also associated with a higher rate of hemoperitoneum and variceal bleeding resulting in a higher mortality rate of 0.7–1.9% [122].

Key Points

- Hepatocellular carcinoma is the fifth most common cause of cancer in the world with increasing incidence and high mortality rate if left untreated.
- The liver is the primary and solitary site of metastatic disease in many malignancies, most commonly colorectal carcinoma.
- Fewer than 20% of cases of patients with metastatic colorectal cancer and hepatocellular carcinoma are candidates for surgical therapy.
- Hepatic ablative techniques have the best outcomes when targeted tumors are 3 cm or smaller.
- Contraindications to percutaneous ablation include: patients with significant extrahepatic disease, Childs class C cirrhosis, active infection, lesions that are inaccessible, tumors that occupy greater than 30% of the liver volume, and tumor proximity of less than 1–2 cm to the main bile ducts.
- The use of preprocedure antibiotics should be reserved for patients with increased risk of developing hepatic abscess postprocedure, such as bacterial colonization of the biliary system and diabetes mellitus.
- An appropriate plan to access the lesion should be determined to avoid damage to other structures. Percutaneous injection of CO_2, dextrose solution, and/or balloon interposition can be used to dissect away adjacent structures and maintain an adequate margin around the ablation probe.
- Most radiofrequency ablation electrodes create an ablation zone of 3 cm, allowing for treatment of a lesion that is 2 cm in diameter with a 5 mm margin. Multiple overlapping ablations or electrodes are needed to treat larger lesions.
- The goal temperature for RFA is 50–100°C.
- Most patients will develop a postablation syndrome consisting of low-grade fever, and muscle aches that should be managed supportively.
- Long-term follow-up after hepatic ablation should be performed with multiphase CT or MRI immediately following treatment as well as 1 and 3 months postprocedure. Once disease control is documented, subsequent follow-up imaging should be performed at 3-month intervals utilizing the same imaging modality for ease of comparison.
- PET scanning and laboratory tumor markers may also be a useful tool to assess for residual or recurrent tumor.
- Microwave ablation is useful for ablation near major hepatic vessels due to the lack of the "heat sink" effect with one study reporting no significant difference between MWA and RFA.
- PEI has higher rates of local tumor progression at the ablation site than RFA. Survival data favors RFA.
- Local control of metastatic disease to the liver such as colorectal carcinoma can be achieved in up to 78% of patients with radiofrequency ablation. Outcomes are best with smaller tumors (<3 cm).
- Survival in patients with metastatic disease is better for patients who are able to undergo surgical resection rather than percutaneous RF ablation.

- Percutaneous ablation can be used for local tumor control in metastatic disease as well as symptomatic relief for patients with metastatic neuroendocrine carcinoma or pain from tumors stretching the hepatic capsule.
- Major complications occur in 0.9–5.7% of patients and include intraperitoneal bleeding, liver abscess, intestinal perforation, pneumothorax/hemothorax, bile duct injury, and seeding of the tract by tumor.
- The mortality rate from hepatic RF ablation is 0.1–0.5%.
- Minor complications or side effects include periprocedural pain, fever, asymptomatic pleural effusion, and grounding pad burns with an overall rate of minor complications ranging from 1.7% to 6.3%.

References

1. Llovet JM, Burroughs A, Bruix J. Hepatocellular carcinoma. Lancet. 2003;362:1907–17.
2. Sherman M. Hepatocellular carcinoma: epidemiology, risk factors, and screening. Semin Liver Dis. 2005;25:143–54.
3. Bruix J, Boix L, Sala M, Llovet JM. Focus on hepatocellular carcinoma. Cancer Cell. 2004;5:215–9.
4. Bruix J, Sherman M. Management of hepatocellular carcinoma. Hepatology. 2005;42:1208–36.
5. Bruix J, Sherman M, Llovet JM, Beaugrand M, Lencioni R, Burroughs AK. Clinical management of hepatocellular carcinoma. Conclusions of the Barcelona-2000 EASL conference. European Association for the Study of the Liver. J Hepatol. 2001;35:421–30.
6. El-Serag HB. Hepatocellular carcinoma: an epidemiologic view. J Clin Gastroenterol. 2002;35:S72–8.
7. Choi TK, Edward CS, Fan ST, Francis PT, Wong J. Results of surgical resection for hepatocellular carcinoma. Hepatogastroenterology. 1990;37:172–5.
8. Franco D, Capussotti L, Smadja C. Resection of hepatocellular carcinomas. Results in 72 European patients with cirrhosis. Gastroenterology. 1990;98:733–8.
9. Llovet JM, Fuster J, Bruix J. Intention-to-treat analysis of surgical treatment for early hepatocellular carcinoma: resection versus transplantation. Hepatology. 1999;30:1434–40.
10. Nagorney DM, van Heerden JA, Ilstrup DM, Adson MA. Primary hepatic malignancy: surgical management and determinants of survival. Surgery. 1989;106:740–8.
11. Tsuzuki T, Sugioka A, Ueda M, et al. Hepatic resection for hepatocellular carcinoma. Hepatic resection for hepatocellular carcinoma. Surgery. 1990;107:511–20.
12. Bruix J, Llovet JM. Prognostic prediction and treatment strategy in hepatocellular carcinoma. Hepatology. 2002;35:519–24.
13. Fong Y, Cohen AM, Fortner JG, et al. Liver resection for colorectal metastases. J Clin Oncol. 1997;15:938–46.
14. Kalva SP, Thabet A, Wicky S. Recent advances in transarterial therapy of primary and secondary liver malignancies. Radiographics. 2008;28:101–17.
15. Abdalla EK, Vauthey JN, Ellis LM, et al. Recurrence and outcomes following hepatic resection, radiofrequency ablation, and combined resection/ablation for colorectal liver metastases. Ann Surg. 2004;239:818–25.
16. Cady B, Jenkins RL, Steele Jr GD, et al. Surgical margin in hepatic resection for colorectal metastasis: a critical and improvable determinant of outcome. Ann Surg. 1998;227:566–71.
17. Choti MA, Sitzmann JV, Tiburi MF, et al. Trends in long-term survival following liver resection for hepatic colorectal metastases. Ann Surg. 2002;235:759–66.

18. Howard JH, Tzeng CW, Smith JK, et al. Radiofrequency ablation for unresectable tumors of the liver. Am Surg. 2008;74:594–600.
19. Kornprat P, Jarnagin WR, Gonen M, et al. Outcome after hepatectomy for multiple (four or more) colorectal metastases in the era of effective chemotherapy. Ann Surg Oncol. 2007; 14:1151–60.
20. Crocetti L, de Baere T, Lencioni R. Quality improvement guidelines for radiofrequency ablation of liver tumours. Cardiovasc Intervent Radiol. 2010;33:11–7.
21. Jansen MC, van Hillegersberg R, Chamuleau RA, van Delden OM, Gouma DJ, van Gulik TM. Outcome of regional and local ablative therapies for hepatocellular carcinoma: a collective review. Eur J Surg Oncol. 2005;31:331–47.
22. McGahan JP, Dodd 3rd GD. Radiofrequency ablation of the liver: current status. Am J Roentgenol. 2001;176:3–16.
23. Bhardwaj N, Strickland AD, Ahmad F, Atanesyan L, West K, Lloyd DM. A comparative histological evaluation of the ablations produced by microwave, cryotherapy and radiofrequency in the liver. Pathology. 2009;41:168–72.
24. Goldberg SN, Gazelle GS, Compton CC, Mueller PR, Tanabe KK. Treatment of intrahepatic malignancy with radiofrequency ablation: radiologic-pathologic correlation. Cancer. 2000; 88:2452–63.
25. Lu DS, Yu NC, Raman SS, et al. Radiofrequency ablation of hepatocellular carcinoma: treatment success as defined by histologic examination of the explanted liver. Radiology. 2005; 234:954–60.
26. McWilliams JP, Yamamoto S, Raman SS, et al. Percutaneous ablation of hepatocellular carcinoma: current status. J Vasc Interv Radiol. 2010;21:S204–13.
27. Livraghi T, Goldberg SN, Lazzaroni S, et al. Hepatocellular carcinoma: radio-frequency ablation of medium and large lesions. Radiology. 2000;214:761–8.
28. de Baere T, Risse O, Kuoch V, et al. Adverse events during radiofrequency treatment of 582 hepatic tumors. Am J Roentgenol. 2003;181:695–700.
29. Raman SS, Aziz D, Chang X, Sayre J, Lassman C, Lu D. Minimizing diaphragmatic injury during radiofrequency ablation: efficacy of intraabdominal carbon dioxide insufflation. Am J Roentgenol. 2004;183:197–200.
30. Song I, Rhim H, Lim HK, Kim YS, Choi D. Percutaneous radiofrequency ablation of hepatocellular carcinoma abutting the diaphragm and gastrointestinal tracts with the use of artificial ascites: safety and technical efficacy in 143 patients. Eur Radiol. 2009;19:2630–40.
31. Yamakado K, Nakatsuka A, Akeboshi M, Takeda K. Percutaneous radiofrequency ablation of liver neoplasms adjacent to the gastrointestinal tract after balloon catheter interposition. J Vasc Interv Radiol. 2003;14:1183–6.
32. Crocetti L, Lencioni R, Debeni S, See TC, Pina CD, Bartolozzi C. Targeting liver lesions for radiofrequency ablation: an experimental feasibility study using a CT-US fusion imaging system. Invest Radiol. 2008;43:33–9.
33. Livraghi T, Benedini V, Lazzaroni S, Meloni F, Torzilli G, Vettori C. Long term results of single session percutaneous ethanol injection in patients with large hepatocellular carcinoma. Cancer. 1998;83:48–57.
34. Livraghi T, Lazzaroni S, Pellicano S, Ravasi S, Torzilli G, Vettori C. Percutaneous ethanol injection of hepatic tumors: single-session therapy with general anesthesia. Am J Roentgenol. 1993;161:1065–9.
35. Lencioni R, Crocetti L, Cioni D, et al. Single-session percutaneous ethanol ablation of early-stage hepatocellular carcinoma with a multipronged injection needle: results of a pilot clinical study. J Vasc Interv Radiol. 2010;21:1533–8.
36. Goldberg SN, Gazelle GS, Mueller PR. Thermal ablation therapy for focal malignancy: a unified approach to underlying principles, techniques, and diagnostic imaging guidance. Am J Roentgenol. 2000;174:323–31.
37. Akriviadis EA, Llovet JM, Efremidis SC, et al. Hepatocellular carcinoma. Br J Surg. 1998; 85:1319–31.

38. Livraghi T, Goldberg SN, Lazzaroni S, Meloni F, Solbiati L, Gazelle GS. Small hepatocellular carcinoma: treatment with radio-frequency ablation versus ethanol injection. Radiology. 1999;210:655–61.
39. Skinner MG, Iizuka MN, Kolios MC, Sherar MD. A theoretical comparison of energy sources – microwave, ultrasound and laser – for interstitial thermal therapy. Phys Med Biol. 1998;43: 3535–47.
40. Dromain C, de Baere T, Elias D, et al. Hepatic tumors treated with percutaneous radio-frequency ablation: CT and MR imaging follow-up. Radiology. 2002;223:255–62.
41. Filippone A, Iezzi R, Di Fabio F, Cianci R, Grassedonio E, Storto ML. Multidetector-row computed tomography of focal liver lesions treated by radiofrequency ablation: spectrum of findings at long-term follow-up. J Comput Assist Tomogr. 2007;31:42–52.
42. Lim HK, Choi D, Lee WJ, Kim SH, Lee SJ, Jang HJ, et al. Hepatocellular carcinoma treated with percutaneous radio-frequency ablation: evaluation with follow-up multiphase helical CT. Radiology. 2001;221:447–54.
43. Nghiem HV, Francis IR, Fontana R, et al. Computed tomography appearances of hypervascular hepatic tumors after percutaneous radiofrequency ablation therapy. Curr Probl Diagn Radiol. 2002;31:105–11.
44. Tsuda M, Majima K, Yamada T, Saitou H, Ishibashi T, Takahashi S. Hepatocellular carcinoma after radiofrequency ablation therapy: dynamic CT evaluation of treatment. Clin Imaging. 2001;25:409–15.
45. Bartolozzi C, Lencioni R, Caramella D, Mazzeo S, Ciancia EM. Treatment of hepatocellular carcinoma with percutaneous ethanol injection: evaluation with contrast-enhanced MR imaging. Am J Roentgenol. 1994;162:827–31.
46. Sironi S, Livraghi T, Meloni F, De Cobelli F, Ferrero C, Del Maschio A. Small hepatocellular carcinoma treated with percutaneous RF ablation: MR imaging follow-up. Am J Roentgenol. 1999;173:1225–9.
47. Vossen JA, Buijs M, Kamel IR. Assessment of tumor response on MR imaging after locoregional therapy. Tech Vasc Interv Radiol. 2006;9:125–32.
48. Donckier V, Van Laethem JL, Goldman S, et al. [F-18] fluorodeoxyglucose positron emission tomography as a tool for early recognition of incomplete tumor destruction after radiofrequency ablation for liver metastases. J Surg Oncol. 2003;84:215–23.
49. Kuehl H, Antoch G, Stergar H, et al. Comparison of FDG-PET, PET/CT and MRI for follow-up of colorectal liver metastases treated with radiofrequency ablation: initial results. Eur J Radiol. 2008;67:362–71.
50. Travaini LL, Trifiro G, Ravasi L, Monfardini L, Della Vigna P, Bonomo G. Role of [18F]FDG-PET/CT after radiofrequency ablation of liver metastases: preliminary results. Eur J Nucl Med Mol Imaging. 2008;35:1316–22.
51. Anderson CD, Vachharajani N, Doyle M, et al. Advanced donor age alone does not affect patient or graft survival after liver transplantation. J Am Coll Surg. 2008;207:847–52.
52. Duffy JP, Hiatt JR, Busuttil RW. Surgical resection of hepatocellular carcinoma. Cancer J. 2008;14:100–10.
53. Fong Y, Sun RL, Jarnagin W, Blumgart LH. An analysis of 412 cases of hepatocellular carcinoma at a Western center. Ann Surg. 1999;229:790–9.
54. Lencioni R, Bartolozzi C, Caramella D. Treatment of small hepatocellular carcinoma with percutaneous ethanol injection. Analysis of prognostic factors in 105 Western patients. Cancer. 1995;76:1737–46.
55. Ebara M, Okabe S, Kita K, Sugiura N, Fukuda H, Yoshikawa M, et al. Percutaneous ethanol injection for small hepatocellular carcinoma: therapeutic efficacy based on 20-year observation. J Hepatol. 2005;43:458–64.
56. Lencioni R, Pinto F, Armillotta N, et al. Long-term results of percutaneous ethanol injection therapy for hepatocellular carcinoma in cirrhosis: a European experience. Eur Radiol. 1997;7:514–9.
57. Livraghi T, Giorgio A, Marin G, et al. Hepatocellular carcinoma and cirrhosis in 746 patients: long-term results of percutaneous ethanol injection. Radiology. 1995;197:101–8.

58. Teratani T, Ishikawa T, Shiratori Y, et al. Hepatocellular carcinoma in elderly patients: beneficial therapeutic efficacy using percutaneous ethanol injection therapy. Cancer. 2002;95:816–23.
59. Khan KN, Yatsuhashi H, Yamasaki K, et al. Prospective analysis of risk factors for early intrahepatic recurrence of hepatocellular carcinoma following ethanol injection. J Hepatol. 2000;32:269–78.
60. Koda M, Murawaki Y, Mitsuda A, et al. Predictive factors for intrahepatic recurrence after percutaneous ethanol injection therapy for small hepatocellular carcinoma. Cancer. 2000;88:529–37.
61. Buscarini L, Buscarini E, Di Stasi M, Vallisa D, Quaretti P, Rocca A. Percutaneous radiofrequency ablation of small hepatocellular carcinoma: long-term results. Eur Radiol. 2001;11:914–21.
62. Cabassa P, Donato F, Simeone F, Grazioli L, Romanini L. Radiofrequency ablation of hepatocellular carcinoma: long-term experience with expandable needle electrodes. Am J Roentgenol. 2006;186:S316–21.
63. Chen MS, Li JQ, Zheng Y, et al. A prospective randomized trial comparing percutaneous local ablative therapy and partial hepatectomy for small hepatocellular carcinoma. Ann Surg. 2006;243:321–8.
64. Choi D, Lim HK, Kim MJ, et al. Recurrent hepatocellular carcinoma: percutaneous radiofrequency ablation after hepatectomy. Radiology. 2004;230:135–41.
65. Choi D, Lim HK, Rhim H, et al. Percutaneous radiofrequency ablation for early-stage hepatocellular carcinoma as a first-line treatment: long-term results and prognostic factors in a large single-institution series. Eur Radiol. 2007;17:684–92.
66. Huang J, Yan L, Cheng Z, et al. A randomized trial comparing radiofrequency ablation and surgical resection for HCC conforming to the milan criteria. Ann Surg. 2010;252:903–12.
67. Lencioni R, Cioni D, Crocetti L, et al. Early-stage hepatocellular carcinoma in patients with cirrhosis: long-term results of percutaneous image-guided radiofrequency ablation. Radiology. 2005;234:961–7.
68. Rossi S, Di Stasi M, Buscarini E, et al. Percutaneous RF interstitial thermal ablation in the treatment of hepatic cancer. Am J Roentgenol. 1996;167:759–68.
69. Shiina S, Tagawa K, Niwa Y, et al. Percutaneous ethanol injection therapy for hepatocellular carcinoma: results in 146 patients. Am J Roentgenol. 1993;160:1023–8.
70. Tateishi R, Shiina S, Teratani T. Percutaneous radiofrequency ablation for hepatocellular carcinoma. An analysis of 1000 cases. Cancer. 2005;103:1201–9.
71. Cho YK, Kim JK, Kim MY, Rhim H, Han JK. Systematic review of randomized trials for hepatocellular carcinoma treated with percutaneous ablation therapies. Hepatology. 2009;49:453–9.
72. Lin SM, Lin CJ, Lin CC, Hsu CW, Chen YC. Radiofrequency ablation improves prognosis compared with ethanol injection for hepatocellular carcinoma < or =4 cm. Gastroenterology. 2004;127:1714–23.
73. Lin SM, Lin CJ, Lin CC, Hsu CW, Chen YC. Randomised controlled trial comparing percutaneous radiofrequency thermal ablation, percutaneous ethanol injection, and percutaneous acetic acid injection to treat hepatocellular carcinoma of 3 cm or less. Gut. 2005;54:1151–6.
74. Orlando A, Leandro G, Olivo M, Andriulli A, Cottone M. Radiofrequency thermal ablation vs. percutaneous ethanol injection for small hepatocellular carcinoma in cirrhosis: meta-analysis of randomized controlled trials. Am J Gastroenterol. 2009;104:514–24.
75. Shiina S, Teratani T, Obi S, et al. A randomized controlled trial of radiofrequency ablation with ethanol injection for small hepatocellular carcinoma. Gastroenterology. 2005;129:122–30.
76. Brunello F, Veltri A, Carucci P, et al. Radiofrequency ablation versus ethanol injection for early hepatocellular carcinoma: A randomized controlled trial. Scand J Gastroenterol. 2008;43:727–35.

77. Lencioni RA, Allgaier HP, Cioni D, et al. Small hepatocellular carcinoma in cirrhosis: randomized comparison of radio-frequency thermal ablation versus percutaneous ethanol injection. Radiology. 2003;228:235–40.
78. Dong B, Liang P, Yu X, et al. Percutaneous sonographically guided microwave coagulation therapy for hepatocellular carcinoma: results in 234 patients. Am J Roentgenol. 2003;180:1547–55.
79. Lu MD, Chen JW, Xie XY, et al. Hepatocellular carcinoma: US-guided percutaneous microwave coagulation therapy. Radiology. 2001;221:167–72.
80. Xu HX, Xie XY, Lu MD, et al. Ultrasound-guided percutaneous thermal ablation of hepatocellular carcinoma using microwave and radiofrequency ablation. Clin Radiol. 2004;59:53–61.
81. Liang P, Dong B, Yu X, et al. Prognostic factors for survival in patients with hepatocellular carcinoma after percutaneous microwave ablation. Radiology. 2005;235:299–307.
82. Shibata T, Iimuro Y, Yamamoto Y, et al. Small hepatocellular carcinoma: comparison of radiofrequency ablation and percutaneous microwave coagulation therapy. Radiology. 2002;223:331–7.
83. Xu KC, Niu LZ, Zhou Q, et al. Sequential use of transarterial chemoembolization and percutaneous cryosurgery for hepatocellular carcinoma. World J Gastroenterol. 2009;15:3664–9.
84. Adam R, Hagopian EJ, Linhares M, et al. A comparison of percutaneous cryosurgery and percutaneous radiofrequency for unresectable hepatic malignancies. Arch Surg. 2002;137:1332–9.
85. Solbiati L, Livraghi T, Goldberg SN, et al. Percutaneous radio-frequency ablation of hepatic metastases from colorectal cancer: long-term results in 117 patients. Radiology. 2001;221:159–66.
86. Gillams AR, Lees WR. Five-year survival following radiofrequency ablation of small, solitary, hepatic colorectal metastases. J Vasc Interv Radiol. 2008;19:712–7.
87. Gillams AR, Lees WR. Five-year survival in 309 patients with colorectal liver metastases treated with radiofrequency ablation. Eur Radiol. 2009;19:1206–13.
88. Jakobs TF, Hoffmann RT, Trumm C, Reiser MF, Helmberger TK. Radiofrequency ablation of colorectal liver metastases: mid-term results in 68 patients. Anticancer Res. 2006;26:671–80.
89. Livraghi T, Solbiati L, Meloni F, Ierace T, Goldberg SN, Gazelle GS. Percutaneous radiofrequency ablation of liver metastases in potential candidates for resection: the "test-of-time approach". Cancer. 2003;97:3027–35.
90. White RR, Avital I, Sofocleous CT, et al. Rates and patterns of recurrence for percutaneous radiofrequency ablation and open wedge resection for solitary colorectal liver metastasis. J Gastrointest Surg. 2007;11:256–63.
91. Gervais DA, Goldberg SN, Brown DB, Soulen MC, Millward SF, Rajan DK. Society of Interventional Radiology position statement on percutaneous radiofrequency ablation for the treatment of liver tumors. J Vasc Interv Radiol. 2009;20:S342–7.
92. Gillams A, Cassoni A, Conway G, Lees W. Radiofrequency ablation of neuroendocrine liver metastases: the Middlesex experience. Abdom Imaging. 2005;30:435–41.
93. Gunabushanam G, Sharma S, Thulkar S, et al. Radiofrequency ablation of liver metastases from breast cancer: results in 14 patients. J Vasc Interv Radiol. 2007;18:67–72.
94. Lawes D, Chopada A, Gillams A, Lees W, Taylor I. Radiofrequency ablation (RFA) as a cytoreductive strategy for hepatic metastasis from breast cancer. Ann R Coll Surg Engl. 2006;88:639–42.
95. Livraghi T, Goldberg SN, Solbiati L, Meloni F, Ierace T, Gazelle GS. Percutaneous radio-frequency ablation of liver metastases from breast cancer: initial experience in 24 patients. Radiology. 2001;220:145–9.
96. Pawlik TM, Vauthey JN, Abdalla EK, Pollock RE, Ellis LM, Curley SA. Results of a single-center experience with resection and ablation for sarcoma metastatic to the liver. Arch Surg. 2006;141:537–43.

97. Mazzaferro V, Regalia E, Doci R, et al. Liver transplantation for the treatment of small hepatocellular carcinomas in patients with cirrhosis. N Engl J Med. 1996;334:693–9.
98. Sauer P, Kraus TW, Schemmer P, et al. Liver transplantation for hepatocellular carcinoma: is there evidence for expanding the selection criteria? Transplantation. 2005;80:S105–8.
99. Yao FY, Ferrell L, Bass NM, et al. Liver transplantation for hepatocellular carcinoma: expansion of the tumor size limits does not adversely impact survival. Hepatology. 2001;33:1394–403.
100. Arii S, Yamaoka Y, Futagawa S, et al. Results of surgical and nonsurgical treatment for small-sized hepatocellular carcinomas: a retrospective and nationwide survey in Japan. The Liver Cancer Study Group of Japan. Hepatology. 2000;32:1224–9.
101. Zhou XD, Tang ZY, Yang BH, et al. Experience of 1000 patients who underwent hepatectomy for small hepatocellular carcinoma. Cancer. 2001;91:1479–86.
102. Abou-Alfa GK, Johnson P, Knox JJ, et al. Doxorubicin plus sorafenib vs doxorubicin alone in patients with advanced hepatocellular carcinoma: a randomized trial. JAMA. 2010;304:2154–60.
103. Llovet JM, Ricci S, Mazzaferro V, et al. Sorafenib in advanced hepatocellular carcinoma. N Engl J Med. 2008;359:378–90.
104. Bharat A, Brown DB, Crippin JS, et al. Pre-liver transplantation locoregional adjuvant therapy for hepatocellular carcinoma as a strategy to improve longterm survival. J Am Coll Surg. 2006;203:411–20.
105. Brown DB, Chapman WC, Cook RD, et al. Chemoembolization of hepatocellular carcinoma: patient status at presentation and outcome over 15 years at a single center. Am J Roentgenol. 2008;190:608–15.
106. Chapman WC, Majella Doyle MB, Stuart JE. Outcomes of neoadjuvant transarterial chemoembolization to downstage hepatocellular carcinoma before liver transplantation. Ann Surg. 2008;248:617–25.
107. Ruutiainen AT, Soulen MC, Tuite CM, et al. Chemoembolization and bland embolization of neuroendocrine tumor metastases to the liver. J Vasc Interv Radiol. 2007;18:847–55.
108. Salem R, Lewandowski RJ, Mulcahy MF, et al. Radioembolization for hepatocellular carcinoma using Yttrium-90 microspheres: a comprehensive report of long-term outcomes. Gastroenterology. 2010;138:52–64.
109. Akahane M, Koga H, Kato N, et al. Complications of percutaneous radiofrequency ablation for hepato-cellular carcinoma: imaging spectrum and management. Radiographics. 2005;25:S57–68.
110. Giorgio A, Tarantino L, de Stefano G, Coppola C, Ferraioli G. Complications after percutaneous saline-enhanced radiofrequency ablation of liver tumors: 3-year experience with 336 patients at a single center. Am J Roentgenol. 2005;184:207–11.
111. Livraghi T, Solbiati L, Meloni MF, Gazelle GS, Halpern EF, Goldberg SN. Treatment of focal liver tumors with percutaneous radio-frequency ablation: complications encountered in a multicenter study. Radiology. 2003;226:441–51.
112. Kim SH, Lim HK, Choi D, et al. Changes in bile ducts after radiofrequency ablation of hepatocellular carcinoma: frequency and clinical significance. Am J Roentgenol. 2004;183:1611–7.
113. Ogawa T, Kawamoto H, Kobayashi Y, et al. Prevention of biliary complication in radiofrequency ablation for hepatocellular carcinoma-Cooling effect by endoscopic nasobiliary drainage tube. Eur J Radiol. 2010;73:385–90.
114. Rhim H, Choi D, Kim YS, Lim HK, Choe BK. Ultrasonography-guided percutaneous radiofrequency ablation of hepatocellular carcinomas: a feasibility scoring system for planning sonography. Eur J Radiol. 2009;75:253–8.
115. Rhim H, Yoon KH, Lee JM, et al. Major complications after radio-frequency thermal ablation of hepatic tumors: spectrum of imaging findings. Radiographics. 2003;23:123–34.
116. Chang IS, Rhim H, Kim SH, et al. Biloma formation after radiofrequency ablation of hepatocellular carcinoma: incidence, imaging features, and clinical significance. Am J Roentgenol. 2010;195:1131–6.

117. Livraghi T, Lazzaroni S, Meloni F, Solbiati L. Risk of tumour seeding after percutaneous radiofrequency ablation for hepatocellular carcinoma. Br J Surg. 2005;92:856–8.
118. Llovet JM, Vilana R, Bru C, et al. Increased risk of tumor seeding after percutaneous radiofrequency ablation for single hepatocellular carcinoma. Hepatology. 2001;33:1124–9.
119. Jaskolka JD, Asch MR, Kachura JR, et al. Needle tract seeding after radiofrequency ablation of hepatic tumors. J Vasc Interv Radiol. 2005;16:485–91.
120. Chopra S, Dodd 3rd GD, Chanin MP, Chintapalli KN. Radiofrequency ablation of hepatic tumors adjacent to the gallbladder: feasibility and safety. Am J Roentgenol. 2003;180:697–701.
121. Di Stasi M, Buscarini L, Livraghi T, et al. Percutaneous ethanol injection in the treatment of hepatocellular carcinoma. A multicenter survey of evaluation practices and complication rates. Scand J Gastroenterol. 1997;32:1168–73.
122. Giorgio A, Tarantino L, de Stefano G, et al. Ultrasound-guided percutaneous ethanol injection under general anesthesia for the treatment of hepatocellular carcinoma on cirrhosis: long-term results in 268 patients. Eur J Ultrasound. 2000;12:145–54.

Chapter 11
Renal Ablation

Nicos Fotiadis

Background

- The incidence of kidney cancer is increasing steadily in the last three decades, with an estimated 60,920 new cases diagnosed in the United States in 2011. The majority of these tumors are small (≤4 cm), organ-confined, and detected incidentally at cross-sectional imaging.
- The current standard of care for clinically localized renal-cell carcinoma (RCC) is surgical, preferably with nephron-sparing surgery (NSS) because of the reported excellent oncologic outcome and overall survival (OS).
- Image-guided ablative techniques, mainly radiofrequency ablation (RFA) and cryoablation, are being used with increased frequency and excellent results in the management of small renal tumors.

Clinical Features/Diagnostic Evaluation

- The classic triad of hematuria, flank pain, and an abdominal mass occurs in less than 10% of patients and is an indication of advanced disease.
- Imaging plays a cardinal role in detection of renal masses. Solid hypo-echoic or mixed echogenicity masses on Ultrasound are highly suspicious for renal cancer and require further evaluation with CT. Well-defined hyper-echoic mass on ultra-

N. Fotiadis, M.D., FRCR
Department of Interventional Oncology, The Royal Marsden NHS Foundation Trust,
Fulham Road, London, SW3 6JJ, UK
e-mail: nicos.fotiadis@rmh.nhs.uk

Department of Interventional Radiology, St Bartholomew's & The Royal London Hospitals,
Whitechapel Road, London, E18 1PD, UK
e-mail: nicos.fotiadis@bartsandthelondon.nhs.uk

T. Clark, T. Sabharwal (eds.), *Interventional Radiology Techniques in Ablation*,
Techniques in Interventional Radiology,
DOI 10.1007/978-0-85729-094-6_11, © Springer-Verlag London 2013

sound are suggestive of angiomyolipoma (AML), which could be confirmed with presence of fat densities on CT.
- Enhancing lesions on CT (>15 Hounsfield units on postcontrast scans) have a 75–80% potential for malignancy. Differentiation between small malignant and benign enhancing lesions on imaging is difficult, with the exception of AMLs, and active surveillance or intervention is required.

Indications

- Small tumors ≤4 cm (T1a). Cryoablation could be used for T1b tumors
- Poor surgical candidates-patients with multiple comorbidities
- Tumor in a solitary kidney
- Bilateral tumors
- Renal insufficiency
- Von-Hippel Lindau disease
- Hereditary form of renal cancer
- Patients preference for ablative management
- Palliation of hematuria

Contraindications

- Irreversible coagulopathy
- Poor life expectancy (<1 year)
- Extensive metastatic disease
- Sepsis
- Pacemaker presence is a relative contraindication for RFA

Patient Preparation

- Patient should be seen in an outpatient clinic by the interventional radiologist and counselled about the procedure; success rates, the associated risks, and the need for long-term imaging follow up.
- Routine clotting studies, (INR < 1.5, platelets > 70,000) and renal function tests preprocedure are required.

Relevant Anatomy

- Exophytic and parenchymal tumors are better treated with RFA because of lack of heat-sink effect from the high-flow central renal vessels.

- Central tumors are associated with higher risk of residual and recurrent tumor due to the heat-sink effect from the high-flow central renal vessels.
- Central tumors are associated with higher risk for injury to the collecting system, and the pyeloperfusion technique is required when treating them with RFA.
- There is some evidence to support the use of cryoablation for central tumors, suggesting higher success rates and less risk of injury to the collecting system.
- Anterior tumors are often too close to thermal energy sensitive structures (bowel, duodenum, pancreas) and the hydrodissection technique is more often required.
- For upper pole tumors, a lateral decubitus position on the treating side decreases the risk of pneumothorax.

Procedure

Sedation/Anesthesia

- RFA could be performed in most cases under conscious sedation provided either by an anesthetist or specialist trained nurse.
- Cryoablation of larger tumors may require insertion of multiple cryoprobes and therefore may be a more prolonged procedure; for this reason, general anesthesia may be helpful in selected cases.
- Lignocaine 1% is used for local anesthesia to the skin and subcutaneous tissues. Bupivacaine 0.25% could be used at the end of the procedure to decrease post-procedure discomfort.

Image Guidance

- CT is the preferred method due to excellent visualization of the anatomy and the relation between needle position, the lesion, and adjacent vital structures. It could also monitor the iceball formation during cryoablation.
- Ultrasound could be used for accurate needle placement in the CT scanner or as a sole image guidance system for posteriorly located exophytic lesions.
- MRI displays the iceball with great accuracy, but needs MRI-combatible systems, which are not commercially available in most centers and whose cost is significantly higher.

Biopsy

- 18-G biopsy before the ablation is required in all cases, with the exception of Von-Hippel Lindau syndrome, heriditary RCCs, and patients with previous renal cancer.

- Biopsy results define the intensity of the subsequent follow-up. No follow-up is required for benign tumors.
- Performing the biopsy at the same session with the ablation is more cost-effective and may be associated with less bleeding and seeding complications due to the ablation of the lesion and the tract after the biopsy.

Technique

- Prone, semiprone, or lateral decubitus position could be used, depending on the location of the lesion. Lateral decubitus, with the treating side down, could reduce the risk of pneumothorax for high upper-pole lesions.
- When a thermal-sensitive structure (colon, duodenum, pancreas, adrenal) is within 1 cm from the target lesion, an adjunctive maneuver is used to create an at least 1-cm plane between the lesion and adjacent sensitive organ.
- *Hydrossicetion* with 5% Dextrose is most commonly used when performing RFA. The RF probe is inserted inside the lesion and subsequently a 22-G spinal needle is inserted between the lesion and the colon. (Fig. 11.1). Fifty milliliter of Dextrose 5% is injected and another CT is performed to check for adequate separation of the structure. Usually, 150–200 ml of dextrose is enough for adequate dissection. Fine needle could stay in place during ablation, for "top-up" with dextrose if needed.
- CO_2 or air could also be used, but not normal saline when performing RFA, because of the theoretical risk of current transimission through the ions of the saline.
- RFA of central lesions abbuting the collecting system and the ureter requires retrograde *pyeloperfusion* with cold dextrose 5% (Fig. 11.2). A 6F ureteric catheter is inserted transurethrally by the urologist and is taped to a folley catheter to prevent its displacement. Cold dextrose 5% is infused during the ablation, usually 1,000–1,500 ml is requited. The ureteric catheter is removed with the conclusion of the procedure.

Endpoint

- The aim of the treatment is the creation of an ablation zone, which involves the renal mass and extends at least 0.5 cm around the lesion.
- When using cryoablation, a double freeze – thaw cycle is required to achieve cell death in the treatment area. The first freeze lasts 8–15 min and the second freeze lasts 5–20 min. Each thaw cycle lasts ~10 min. Mean treatment time is ~40 min.

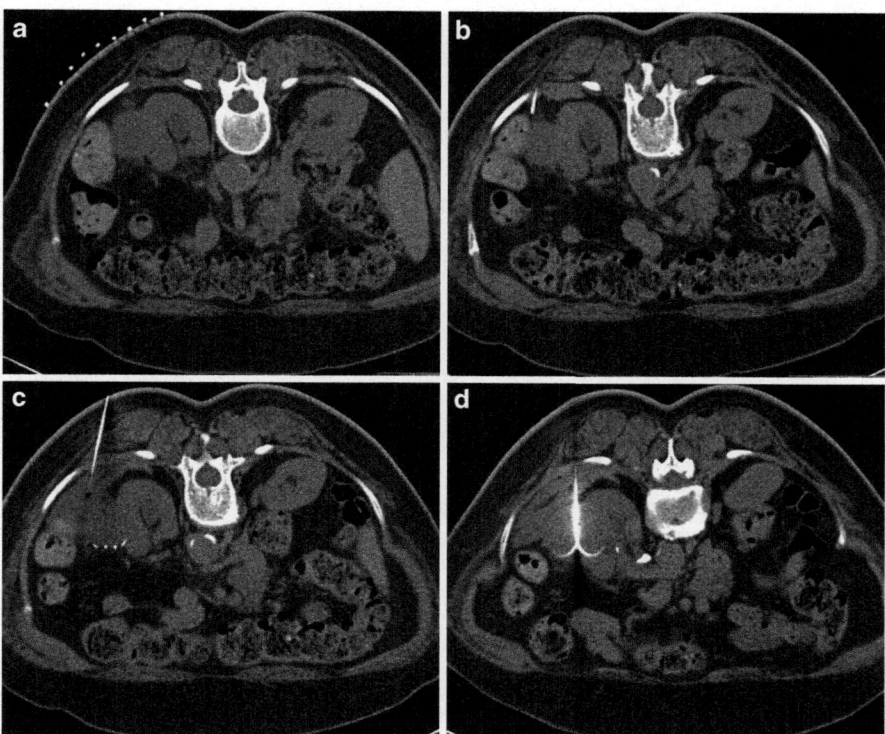

Fig. 11.1 (**a**) Ascending colon is noted adjacent to the large 4 cm right mid-pole renal tumor. (**b**) A 22-G spinal needle is inserted adjacent to the tumor and the colon and 5% Dextrose is injected. (**c**) With the spinal needle still in place, the RF probe is inserted inside the lesion. (**d**) Ablation could start when an adequate 1-cm plane between the mass and the colon is achieved

- When using RFA, we are aiming to create a temperature >60° and <105° inside the ablation zone. This is achieved by either measuring the temperature itself (e.g. Starburst electrode, RITA Medical systems, Mountain view, CA, USA) or the impedance (e.g. Leveen Electrode, Boston Scientific, Watertown, MA, USA), or both (Cool-tip electrode, Covidien, Boulder, CO, USA).

Immediate Postprocedure Care

- Young fit patients could have the procedure as daycase and be discharged in the evening after 6 h of uneventful follow-up.
- Majority of the patients will need an overnight stay in the hospital.

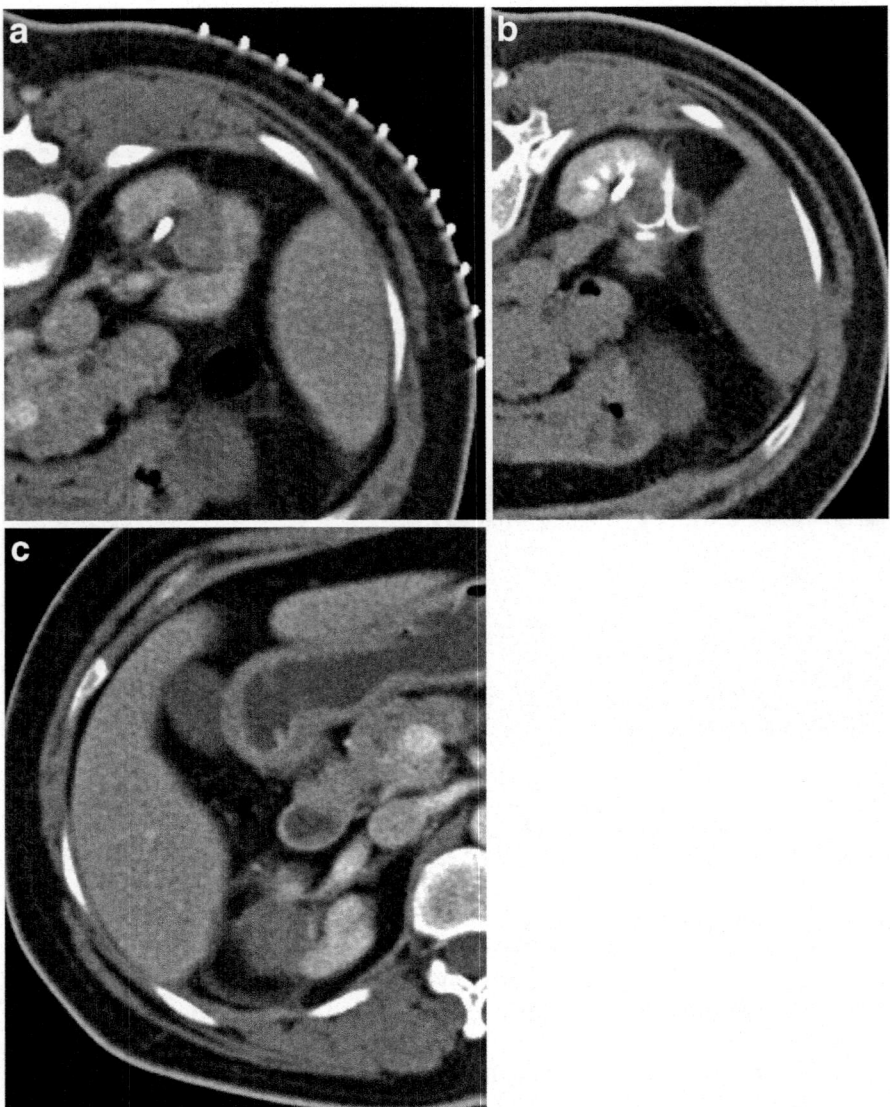

Fig. 11.2 (**a**) Central 2.2-cm tumor abutting the collecting system. 6F ureteric catheter has been inserted and noted next to lesion. (**b**) The RF probe is inserted and cool perfusion of the collecting system with Dextrose 5% starts. (**c**) Follow-up CT at 6 months showing complete ablation of the tumor

Follow up

- Pre and post contrast-enhanced CT scan at 6 weeks, 6 months, 12 months, and yearly after that.

- Outpatient appointment, chest x-ray, liver and kidney function tests at 6 weeks, 6 months, and yearly after that.
- Incomplete ablation is defined as any enhancement within the tumor ablation zone on CT or MRI on the initial 6-week imaging after RFA.
- Recurrence is defined as any enhancement or increase in size of the tumor ablation zone, after an initial nonenhancing 6-weeks CT or MRI. These patients are given the option of a repeat ablation or extirpative surgery.

Results

- Medium terms results regarding the oncological efficacy of both RFA and cryoablation are comparable with extirpative surgery. Robust long-term data is still awaited.
- A meta-analysis of 47 studies (nonrandomized comparative studies and case series) including a total of 1,375 tumors treated by RFA ($n = 775$) or cryoablation ($n = 600$) reported local tumor progression (defined as radiographic or pathological evidence of residual disease after initial treatment, regardless of time to recurrence) in 13% (100/775) and 5% (31/600) of tumors, respectively, at a mean 19-month follow-up ($p < 0.001$). The meta-analysis reported progression to metastatic disease in 2% (19/775) of tumors treated by RFA and 1% (6/600) of tumors treated by cryoablation ($p =$ not significant).

Alternative Therapies

- Partial nephrectomy is still the standard of care for patients with stage T1a renal cancer.
- There is an argument for active surveillance of small renal masses in unfit patients or with limited life expectancy. These patients though need to be counselled about the small but not negligible risk of tumor progression, possible loss of oportunity of nephron sparing intervention and lack of curative treatment if metastatic disease develops.

Complications

- Hemorrhage is reported in approximately 5% of patients, with a need for tranfusion in 1% and need for embolization <1%. Hemorrhagic complications are slightly more common with cryoablation, since blood vessels are not cauterized as with RFA.

Key Points
- The ideal renal tumor for the percutaneous approach is small (<3 cm), partially exophytic, and posteriorly located in a patient who cannot tolerate a partial nephrectomy.
- Percutaneous RFA is a faster and less-expensive procedure than percutaneous cryoablation. Cryoablation is potentially more effective in central and larger lesions.
- Hydrodissection and pyeloperfusion techniques could prevent injuries to the adjacent organs and the collecting system.
- Close follow-up is required, with low threshold for re-intervention.

- Injury to the collecting system (ureteric stricture, urine leak) is seen in ~1–2% of patients and could be prevented with the pyeloperfusion technique. There is less risk of injury to the collecting system with Cryo.
- Injury to the bowel could be serious, but luckily is seen in less than 1% of patients. Hydrodissection with dextrose 5% could prevent bowel injuries.
- Pain and paresthesias at the puncture site are the most common self-limited complications.

Suggested Reading

Fotiadis NI, Sabharwal T, Morales JP, et al. Combined percutaneous radiofrequency ablation and ethanol injection of renal tumours: midterm results. Eur Urol. 2007;52(3):777–84.

Gervais DA, McGovern FJ, Arelano RS, McDougal WS, Mueller PR. Radiofrequency ablation of renal cell carcinoma, part I. Indications, results and role in patient management over a six-year period and ablation of 100 tumours. AJR Am J Roentgenol. 2005;185:64–71.

Knuckle DA, Egleton BL, Uzzo RG. Excise, ablate or observe: the small renal mass dilemma – a meta-analysis and review. J Urol. 2008;179:1227–34.

Rosenberg MD, Kim CY, Tsivian M, et al. Percutaneous cryoablation of renal lesions with radiographic ice ball involvement of the renal sinus: analysis of hemorrhagic and collecting system complications. AJR Am J Roentgenol. 2011;196(4):935–9.

Van Poppel H, Becker F, Caddedu JA, et al. Treatment of localized renal cell carcinoma. Eur Urol. 2011;60(4):662–72.

Chapter 12
Adrenal Ablation: Primary Tumors and Metastatic Disease

Michael D. Beland and William W. Mayo-Smith

Clinical Features

- Adrenal neoplasms are common, estimated to occur in approximately 1% of the general population.
- Adrenal tumors represent a diverse group of neoplasms that can be separated into primary versus metastatic disease.
- The most common adrenal neoplasm is a nonfunctioning adenoma, which is usually discovered incidentally on cross-sectional imaging examinations.
- Primary neoplasms of the adrenal gland include nonfunctioning or cortisol-producing adenomas, adrenal cortical carcinomas, pheochromocytomas, and aldosteronomas.
- Primary adrenal cortical carcinoma is a rare tumor originating in the adrenal cortex and up to 40–70% of patients have metastases at the time of diagnosis.
- Adrenal cortical carcinomas do not respond well to chemotherapy or radiation therapy and surgery has been the primary preferred method of treatment.
- Pheochromocytoma is a rare tumor originating in the chromaffin cells of the adrenal medulla.
- Generally, the treatment for functioning adrenal neoplasms and adrenal cortical carcinoma is surgical resection.
- The adrenal gland is a common site of metastases and metastasis to the adrenal gland is the most common malignant adrenal neoplasm.
- Lung carcinoma is the most common primary tumor that metastasizes to the adrenal gland.
- Other primary tumors with a propensity to metastasize to the adrenal gland include renal cell carcinoma, gastrointestinal tumors, and melanoma.

M.D. Beland, M.D. • W.W. Mayo-Smith, M.D. (✉)
Department of Diagnostic Imaging, Rhode Island Hospital, The Warren Alpert Medical School of Brown University, 593 Eddy Street, Providence, RI 02903, USA
e-mail: mbeland@lifespan.org; wmayo-smith@lifespan.org

T. Clark, T. Sabharwal (eds.), *Interventional Radiology Techniques in Ablation*,
Techniques in Interventional Radiology,
DOI 10.1007/978-0-85729-094-6_12, © Springer-Verlag London 2013

- Although controversial, isolated adrenal metastatic disease can be treated by surgical resection.
- Less-invasive techniques to treat adrenal neoplasms have been used including percutaneous chemical ablation through the injection of alcohol or acetic acid, radiofrequency ablation (RFA), and cryoablation.

Diagnostic Evaluation

Clinical

- In patients without a primary malignancy, the vast majority of incidentally detected adrenal masses are benign.
- The primary objective in managing adrenal neoplasms is differentiating nonfunctioning adenomas from malignant or biochemically active adrenal tumors.
- Incidental nonfunctioning adenomas are benign, do not affect patient survival, and do not require treatment.
- A functioning adenoma can be identified through correlation with history, physical examination, and appropriate biochemical work-up.
- Pheochromocytomas are hormonally active and produce excessive catecholamines leading to hypertension, headaches, diaphoresis, tachycardia, and anxiety.
- Aldosterone-secreting adrenal cortical adenoma results in excessive secretion of aldosterone causing secondary hypertension, metabolic alkalosis, and hypokalemia.
- It is estimated that primary hyperaldosteronism is the causative factor in less than 1% of patients with hypertension.

Laboratory

- Biochemical work-up of an adrenal adenoma should be performed to assess functional status.
- Laboratory tests ordered may be tailored depending on the presence or absence of clinical symptoms.
- Biochemical tests ordered for aldosteronoma include plasma aldosterone concentration and plasma renin activity (after the patient has been upright for at least 2 h).
- Initial screening for a cortisol-producing adenoma is a low-dose dexamethasone suppression test.
- Biochemical evaluation for a pheochromocytoma generally includes measuring serum metanephrines and, if necessary, a 24-h urine collection for catecholamines, vanillylmandelic acid, and metanephrines.

Imaging

- Because of the increasing use of cross-sectional imaging, adrenal masses are commonly detected, with reported frequency of up to 5% at abdominal CT.
- Imaging for diagnosis of pheochromocytoma should only be performed if there are biochemical abnormalities identified by serum or urine testing.
- Aldosteronomas are unilateral in the vast majority of cases. They are small and difficult to detect on cross-sectional imaging, with over 20% being less than 1 cm.
- In a patient with a known primary malignancy, imaging may detect an indeterminate adrenal mass, which can be further evaluated with dedicated adrenal mass protocol CT, MRI, PET, or biopsy.
- Adrenal adenomas commonly have high intracellular lipid and rapid wash out of intravenous contrast when compared to metastases.
- A dedicated adrenal mass protocol CT relies on two different properties of the adrenal mass: intracellular lipid, which determines the density of the mass, and perfusion, which is calculated by intravenous contrast washout.
- Adrenal MRI uses chemical-shift artifact to identify the high lipid content of adrenal adenomas.
- PET will show if a tumor is metabolically active suggesting it is more likely to be metastatic although some adrenal adenomas may show uptake on F-18 FDG PET.
- In the case of indeterminate imaging work-up or a high clinical suspicion of an adrenal metastasis, biopsy can be performed, generally under CT-guidance.

Indications/Contraindications

Patient Preparation

- All patients should be seen in advance of the procedure to determine whether they are appropriate candidates for ablative therapy and to explain the procedure in detail and answer questions.
- All patients should have a staging CT of the chest, abdomen, and pelvis before undergoing ablation of an adrenal mass.
- The adrenal glands are biochemically active organs, which serve as a storage depot for several potent steroid hormones and catecholamines.
- Performing adrenal ablation carries a significant risk of releasing a large amount of these hormones rapidly into the bloodstream.
- The release of catecholamines can be especially problematic causing rapid increase in heart rate and blood pressure during the procedure.
- While this may not happen every time, the risk is substantial enough to warrant pretreatment alpha and beta blockade, which will be discussed below in further detail.

Relevant Anatomy

Normal Anatomy

- Located between the upper poles of the kidneys and the diaphragm.
- The adrenal gland is within the perinephric fat deep to the renal capsule.
- Normal adrenal gland has two limbs meeting to form an inverted "Y" on axial plane imaging.
- The thickness of each limb should be less than 6 mm.
- The outer cortex of the adrenal gland is the zona glomerulosa, responsible for aldosterone production.
- The inner cortex contains the zona fasiculata responsible for cortisol production and the zona reticularis responsible for sex hormone production.
- The medulla is responsible for adrenergic hormone production.
- Arterial supply is generally supplied by superior, middle, and inferior adrenal arteries arising from the inferior phrenic artery, aorta, and renal artery, respectively.
- Two thirds of patients will have a single right adrenal vein draining into the IVC.
- Left adrenal vein almost always drains into the left renal vein.

Aberrant Anatomy

- There may be only a single arterial source (inferior phrenic, renal, or aorta) in 5% of people.
- Up to 10% of patients will have an accessory right adrenal gland vein draining into a common trunk with an accessory right hepatic vein.
- Ectopic adrenal tissue can occur anywhere along the embryonic urogenital ridge.

Equipment

- RFA is one of the most widely applied methods of thermal ablation and has been well established as a safe and effective treatment option for many solid malignancies (Fig. 12.1).
- RFA works by transforming radiofrequency energy into heat, which is deposited into the tumor.
- Cryoablation may be used causing tumor necrosis through rapid cell freezing (Fig. 12.2).
- Chemical ablation, which is performed by image-guided instillation of a chemical agent, has largely been replaced by RFA in the United States.

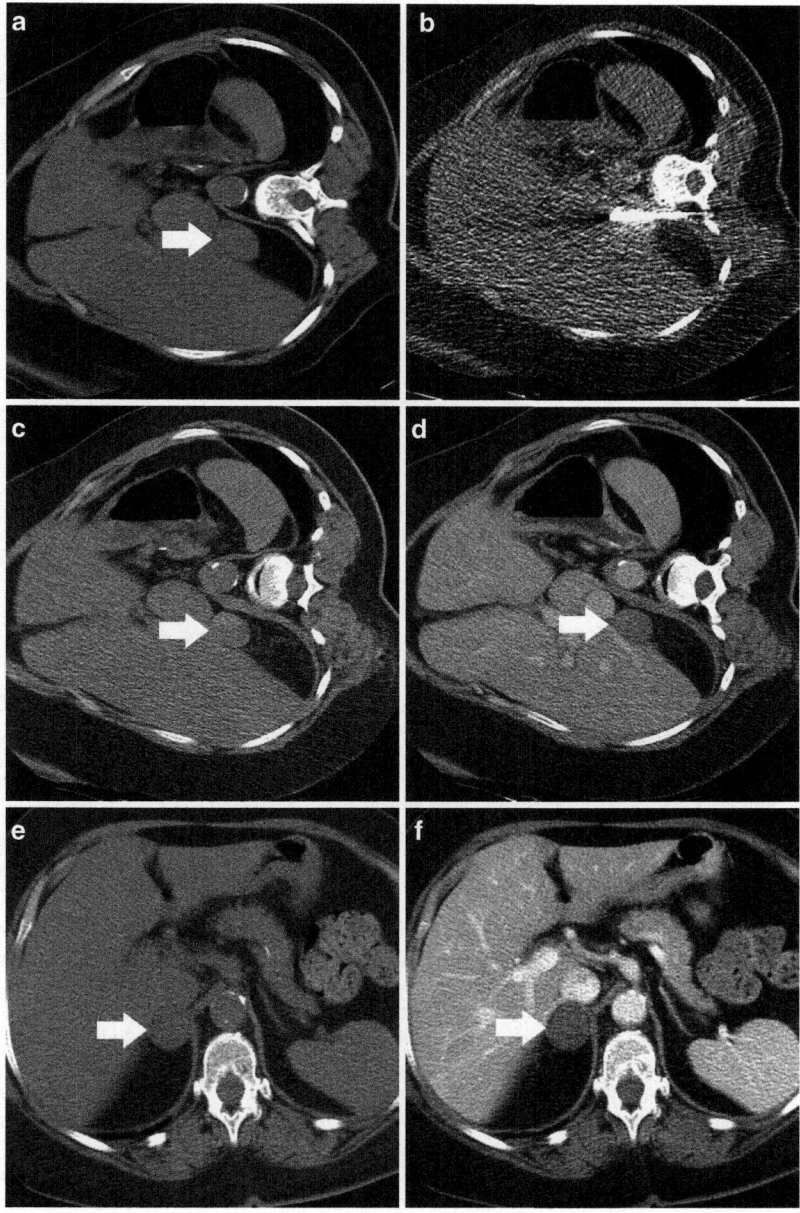

Fig. 12.1 A 54-year-old female with a history of systemic lupus erythromatosis, coronary artery disease with coronary stents who is status post left nephrectomy for renal-cell carcinoma 2 years ago. She now presents with an isolated right adrenal metastasis. Radiofrequency ablation was performed using a cluster electrode with alpha and beta blockade. (**a**) CT image obtained for planning of electrode placement in the right lateral decubitus position demonstrates right adrenal metastasis (*arrow*). (**b**) Portion of the cluster electrode is visible in the tumor. (**c**) Noncontrast CT, and (**d**) intravenous contrast-enhanced CT performed on the same day following RFA shows no evidence of enhancement of the tumor (*arrows*). (**e**) Noncontrast and (**f**) intravenous contrast-enhanced CT performed 5 years after RFA shows persistent nonenhancement of treated tumor (*arrows*) with no evidence of local recurrence

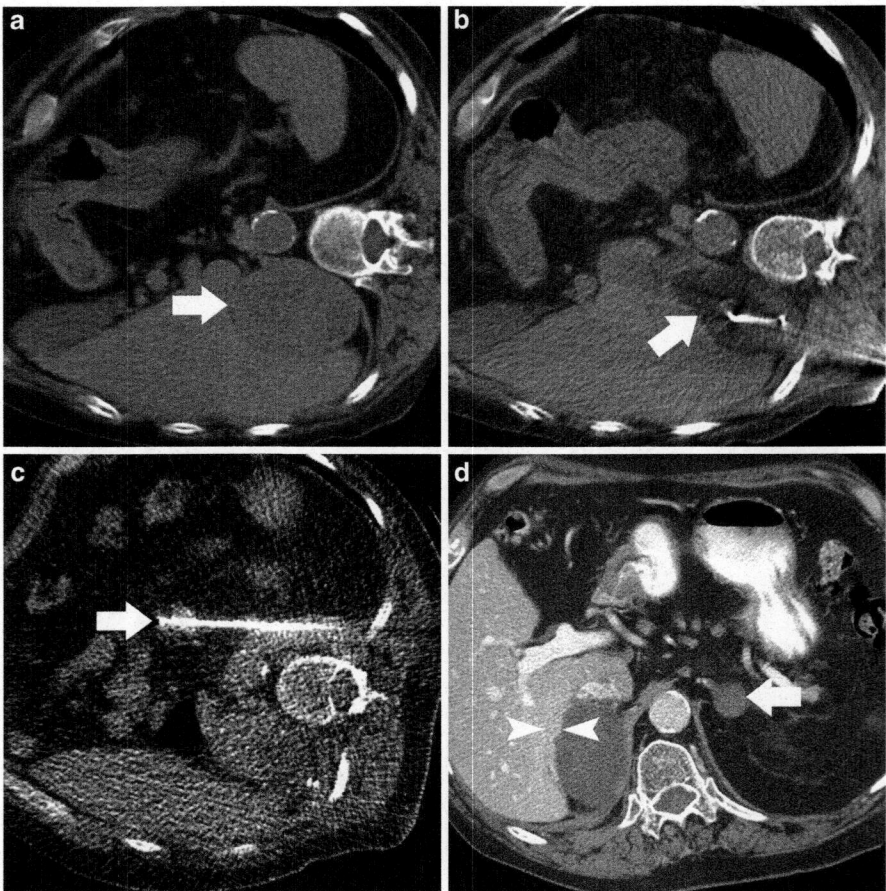

Fig. 12.2 A 69-year-old male with history of renal-cell carcinoma, status post right nephrectomy with adrenal metastases. A right adrenal metastasis was previously ablated with RFA 3 years ago and the patient now presents with a large 8-cm recurrence in the right adrenal gland and a new 1.5-cm left adrenal metastasis. Cryoablation was chosen to treat the right metastasis due to large size with subsequent RFA of the left metastasis 2 months later. (**a**) Preprocedural right lateral decubitus CT image demonstrates right adrenal metastases (*arrow*). (**b**) Right lateral decubitus CT image during cryoablation of the right adrenal metastasis shows 1 of the 7 cryoapplicators used in the procedure. Note the low density ice ball surrounding the applicator (*arrow*). (**c**) Right lateral decubitus CT image during RFA of the left adrenal metastasis shows electrode in lesion (*arrow*). (**d**) Axial contrast-enhanced CT image obtained 1 month after RFA shows complete nonenhancement of the left adrenal metastasis (*arrow*) and near complete necrosis of the right adrenal metastasis with a lateral rim of residual enhancing tumor (between *arrowheads*)

- The most common chemical agent used for tumor ablation is ethanol, although other agents such as acetic acid have been used.
- Microwave ablation and laser interstitial photocoagulation may become more widely applied in the future but are not commonly used currently.

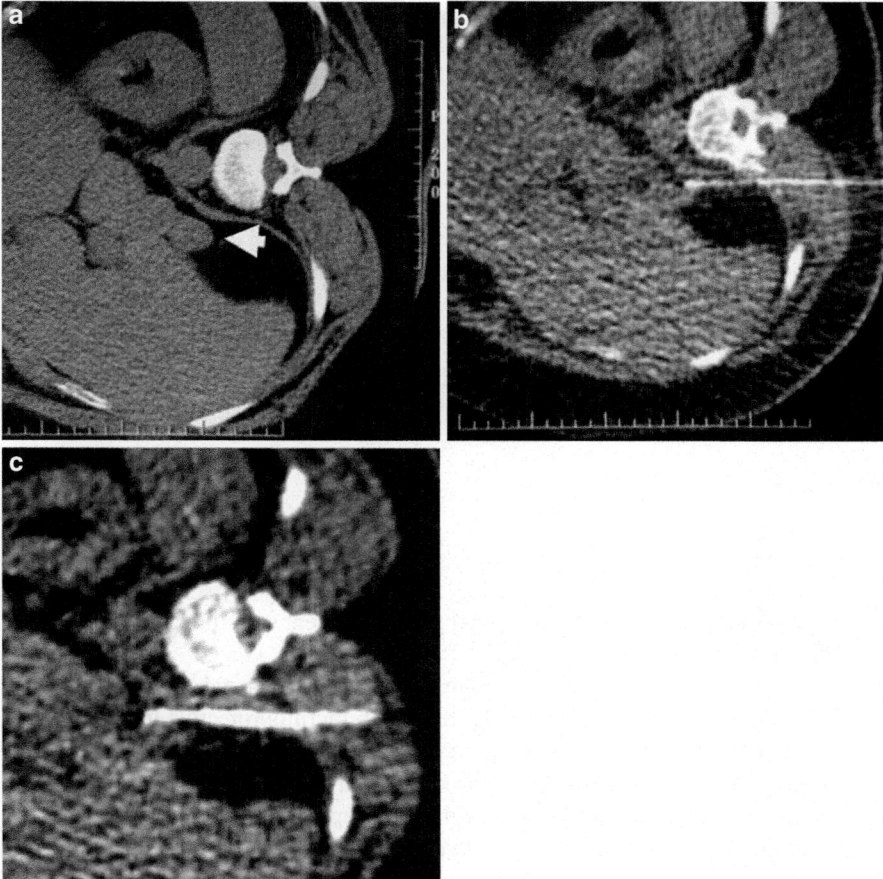

Fig. 12.3 A 68-year-old male with elevated serum metanephrines and elevated chromogranin A levels with a right adrenal mass. He was premedicated with alpha and beta blockade for 5 weeks prior to procedure. (**a**) Right lateral decubitus image demonstrating right adrenal mass suspicious for pheochromocytoma (*arrow*). (**b**) Right lateral decubitus image demonstrating biopsy needle in adrenal mass. Biopsy results were positive for pheochromocytoma. (**c**) Right lateral decubitus image demonstrating cluster RFA electrode during ablation of the the right adrenal pheochromocytoma.

Preprocedure Medications

- Most interventional radiologists perform adrenal ablations with alpha and beta blockade. Appropriate blockade is commonly administered by a referring endocrinologist.
- Patients undergoing percutaneous ablation of a pheochromocytoma should always undergo alpha and beta blockade (Fig. 12.3).
- There is no way to distinguish which patients will be at risk for a hypertensive crisis prior to the procedure and there are case reports of patients having hypertensive crises during heating of normal adrenal glands.

- Alpha blockade is accomplished by premedication with phenoxybenzamine for several days prior to the procedure.
- Many patients may also require beta blockade due to the resultant tachycardia associated with alpha blockade.
- It is critical that beta blockade only be performed after adequate alpha blockade because unopposed alpha receptor stimulation can precipitate a hypertensive crisis.
- Sedation can either be given by an anesthesiologist using continuous blood pressure monitoring by an arterial line or using conscious sedation with intravenous midazolam and fentanyl.
- We do not routinely use intravenous or oral antibiotics before or during the ablation procedure.

Procedure

Planning an Access Route

- Because of the location of the adrenal gland, adjacent structures can be at risk of collateral thermal injury.
- The stomach, kidney, pancreas, and liver are at particular risk.
- To isolate the adrenal gland during treatment, thermoprotective techniques can be utilized to displace adjacent structures.
- Specifically, a technique termed hydrodissection can be performed where a catheter is placed adjacent to the adrenal gland through which a 5% dextrose solution is instilled until displacement of critical adjacent structures is adequate to allow safe treatment. We opacify the dextrose solution with 30 cc intravenous contrast per liter of dextrose solution. (It is important not to use saline solutions for hydrodissection as saline can conduct RF current.)
- In general, we prefer to keep the patient in the ipsilateral decubitus position with the treated adrenal gland in the dependent position. This minimizes respiratory excursion and prevents transpulmonary access to the adrenal gland. The dependent lung tends to lose volume increasing access to the dependent adrenal.
- For large adrenal lesions, placing the patient in the prone position can provide a safe access route.

Performing the Procedure

- CT or CT fluoroscopic guidance is the imaging modality of choice for performing percutaneous adrenal ablations because it visualizes the adrenal gland, the applicator, and critical adjacent structures.
- Ultrasound does not reliably image the adrenal nor accurately confirm placement of the treatment applicator within the tumor. In addition, gas production at the

radiofrequency electrode tip can obscure the adrenal lesion under ultrasound guidance.

- MR imaging guidance can be used for this procedure depending on electrode MR compatibility and local institutional practices.
- Different configurations of RFA electrodes can be used depending on the manufacturer and user preference. We prefer the cluster electrode in all lesions as the area of tumor necrosis is larger than a single electrode, requiring fewer applications per patient visit.
- RFA treatment time of approximately 8 min is adequate to induce tumor necrosis with posttreatment intratumoral temperatures measured at the electrode tip exceeding 50°C.
- Larger tumors require multiple applications depending on ablation applicators and configurations used.
- If multiple applications are performed in one adrenal lesion, shorter application times can be used, although it is necessary to confirm adequate treatment by measuring intratumoral temperatures at the end of each application.
- Cryoablation can obtain temperatures from −80°C to less than −150°C. Freezing is accomplished by placement of 1–8 applicators into the tumor depending on tumor size. A treatment consists of two 10-min freezes, each followed by 8-min thaw cycles.
- One of the advantages of cryoablation compared to RFA is that the zone of cell death can be visualized at the time of treatment through visualization of the ice ball on CT.
- Chemical ablation can be performed by either direct percutaneous injection of an agent into the adrenal gland or embolization via the adrenal artery.
- Percutaneous chemical ablation in the adrenal gland can be performed using a small (19–22 gauge) needle or similar-sized lateral side-hole needle into the center of smaller tumors. Larger tumors may require the placement of 2 or 3 needles evenly spaced through the tumor.
- Early reports of chemical ablation in the adrenal gland also described intra-arterial administration of ethanol through catheters placed in the ipsilateral adrenal artery.
- A contrast-enhanced CT exam can be performed immediately after the ablation before the patient is moved from the CT gantry to ensure complete necrosis of the treated adrenal tumor.

Immediate Postprocedure Care

- Postprocedure, patient should be observed in a monitored recovery area for several hours, then discharged home with a family member.
- Oral nonsteroidal anti-inflammatory medications are the mainstay of analgesia after the procedure.
- Oral narcotics can be prescribed but will be needed in less than 50% of patients.

Follow-up and Postprocedure Medications

- Follow-up imaging with a contrast-enhanced CT or MR at 6-month intervals for approximately 2 years after the treatment should be performed to ensure complete tumor destruction.
- Adequate tumor treatment is defined by a decrease in size of the treated adrenal mass or lack of enhancement with intravenous contrast on follow-up imaging with CT or MR (Fig. 12.1).
- Monitoring of biochemical profiles should be performed following ablation of functioning tumors.
- In successfully treated lesions, serum hormone levels generally normalize by 1 week.
- Serum potassium levels should be followed closely after aldosteronoma ablation.
- In patients treated for aldosteronoma or pheochromocytoma, antihypertensive medications should be continued immediately following the procedure and can be gradually tapered as tolerated by the endocrinologist.

Results

- Complete tumor necrosis after a single treatment session is seen in 85% of adrenal tumors treated with RFA.
- RFA of small functional adrenal neoplasms has been successful with all patients having resolution of abnormal biochemical markers after ablation and resolution of clinical symptoms or syndromes, including hypertension and hypokalemia (in patients with aldosteronoma), Cushing syndrome (in the patient with cortisol-secreting tumor), virilizing symptoms (in the patient with testosterone-secreting tumor), and hypertension (in the patient with pheochromocytoma).
- Cryoablation has successfully treated 92% of adrenal metastases.
- Patients premedicated with the α-blocker phenoxybenzamine appear to have a reduced risk of hypertensive crisis during the thaw phase of cryoablation.
- Percutaneous ethanol injection has not gained widespread popularity in the United States.
- The largest ethanol ablation series in the literature reports a complete response rate of 92.3% and a partial response rate of 7.7%. Success was decreased for metastases, with a complete response rate of 30% and partial response rate of 70% 24 months after therapy.
- The standard treatment for adrenal cortical carcinoma remains surgery. However, RFA may be effective at local control of both recurrent adrenal cortical carcinoma as well as metastasis from adrenal cortical carcinoma.

Alternative Therapies

- The traditional treatment of primary adrenal neoplasms includes open and laparoscopic resection.
- Surgical complication rates are approximately 25–28% with laparoscopic resection and 11% with open adrenalectomy.
- Potential complications include bleeding, associated organ injury (mostly splenic), wound complications, cardiac complications (postsurgery myocardial infarction and/or angina), and infectious complications.
- Chemotherapy with mitotane and radiation therapy (particularly for malignant lesions) have been used in an attempt to achieve endocrinologic normalization with less morbidity; however, these have had no significant effect on disease morbidity.

Complications

How to Avoid

- Alpha and beta adrenergic blockade should be considered in all patients to avoid a hypertensive crisis.
- Close intraprocedural monitoring of blood pressure to detect blood pressure elevation as early as possible and be prepared to intervene pharmacologically.
- Ipsilateral treatment side down decubitus positioning to minimize risk of pneumothorax.
- Consider hydrodissection technique to displace adjacent structures, such as spleen, liver, kidney, pancreas, and bowel.

Key Points
- Adrenal tumors represent a heterogeneous group of neoplasms with widely varying prognosis and recommended medical treatments.
- Benign nonfunctioning adenomas require no treatment.
- The precise role of percutaneous ablation in the treatment of neoplasms has yet to be determined.
- In general, adrenal tumors, which may be considered for surgical resection, would also be considered for image-guided ablation.
- Image-guided minimally invasive therapy has an advantage over surgery with its attendant risks as well as increased cost and the necessity for general anesthesia.

- To date, the largest experience has been with RFA of primary and second-ary adrenal neoplasms.
- Further prospective trials comparing RFA with traditional therapies as well as chemical ablation and cryoablation are necessary to further define its role.
- Perhaps, the greatest potential for adrenal tumor ablation lies in the treat-ment of (1) recurrent disease, (2) small biochemically active tumors, and (3) isolated adrenal metastases in appropriate candidates.

Suggested Reading

Brook OR, Mendiratta-Lala M, Brennan D, Siewert B, Faintuch S, Goldberg SN. Imaging findings after radiofrequency ablation of adrenal tumors. AJR Am J Roentgenol. 2011;196(2):382–8.

Inoue H, Nakajo M, Miyazono N, Nishida H, Ueno K, Hokotate H. Transcatheter arterial ablation of aldosteronomas with high-concentration ethanol: preliminary and long-term results. AJR Am J Roentgenol. 1997;168:1241–5.

Maki DD, Haskal ZJ, Matthies A, Langer J, Nisenbaum HL, Vaughn D, Alavi A. Percutaneous ethanol ablation of an adrenal tumor. Am J Roentgenol. 2000;174:1031–2.

Mayo-Smith WW, Dupuy DE. CT guided radiofrequency ablation of adrenal neoplasms: prelimi-nary results. Radiology. 2004;231:225–30.

Mendiratta-Lala M, Brennan DD, Brook OR, Faintuch S, Mowschenson PM, Sheiman RG, Goldberg SN. Efficacy of radiofrequency ablation in the treatment of small functional adrenal neoplasms. Radiology. 2011;258(1):308–16.

Munver R, Del Pizzo JJ, Sosa RE. Adrenal-preserving minimally invasive surgery: the role of laparoscopic partial adrenalectomy, cryosurgery, and radiofrequency ablation of the adrenal gland. Curr Urol Rep. 2003;4:87–92.

Pacek K, Fojo T, Goldstein DS, et al. Radiofrequency ablation (RFA): a novel approach for the treatment of metastatic pheochromocytoma. J Natl Cancer Inst. 2001;93:648–9.

Sudheendra D, Wood BJ. Appropriate premedication risk reduction during adrenal ablation. J Vasc Interv Radiol. 2006;17(8):1367–8 [comment].

Welch BT, Atwell TD, Nichols DA, Wass CT, Callstrom MR, Leibovich BC, Carpenter PC, Mandrekar JN, Charboneau JW. Percutaneous image-guided adrenal cryoablation: procedural considerations and technical success. Radiology. 2011;258(1):301–7.

Wood BJ, Abraham J, Hvizda JL, Alexander HR, Fojo T. Radiofrequency ablation of adrenal tumors and adrenocortical carcinoma metastases. Cancer. 2003;97(3):554–60.

Xiao YY, Tian JL, Li JK, Yang L, Zhang JS. CT-guided percutaneous chemical ablation of adrenal neoplasms. Am J Roentgenol. 2008;190:105–10.

Chapter 13
Prostate Ablation

Georgia Tsoumakidou, Hervé Lang, and Afshin Gangi

Introduction

Prostate cancer (PCa) is the most prevalent cancer in men and among the three first leading causes of cancer death in both American and European men [1, 2]. PCa affects elderly men more often than young men and thus is a major health problem in the developed countries where the proportion of elderly men is high [3].

G. Tsoumakidou, M.D. (✉)
Department of Interventional Radiology, University Hospital of Strasbourg,
1, place de l'Hopital BP 426, Strasbourg 67091, France

Department of Non-vascular Interventional Radiology, University Hospital of Strasbourg,
Strasbourg, France

Department of Urology, University Hospital of Strasbourg,
Strasbourg, France
e-mail: gtsoumakidou@yahoo.com

H. Lang, M.D., Ph.D.
Department of Urology, University Hospital of Strasbourg,
Strasbourg, France

A. Gangi, M.D., Ph.D.
Department of Interventional Radiology, University Hospital of Strasbourg,
1, place de l'Hopital BP 426, Strasbourg, 67091, France

Department of Non-vascular Interventional Radiology, University Hospital of Strasbourg,
Strasbourg, France
e-mail: gangi@rad6.u-strasbg.fr

T. Clark, T. Sabharwal (eds.), *Interventional Radiology Techniques in Ablation*,
Techniques in Interventional Radiology,
DOI 10.1007/978-0-85729-094-6_13, © Springer-Verlag London 2013

Clinical Features

Hereditary factors and the increasing age are important in determining the risk of developing clinical PCa, while several different exogenous factors (food and alcohol consumption, pattern of sexual behavior) also play an important role.

Diagnosis

The diagnosis of PCa is made based on the:

1. Digital rectal examination
2. Level of Prostate Specific Antigen (PSA-level)
3. Transrectal US
4. Prostate MRI
5. Prostate biopsy

The definite diagnosis of PCa depends on findings of prostate adenocarcinoma cells on biopsy cores or surgical specimens. Furthermore, the histopathological examination allows the grading and the determination of the extent of the tumor.

Staging

- Local staging of PCa is done based on the findings of pelvic MRI (dynamic contrast-enhanced MRI and MR-spectroscopy) [4]. The number-sites of positive biopsies, the tumor grade, and the level of serum PSA also play a role on local staging.
- Lymph node staging and the evaluation for metastasis is based on the results of CT-scan and bone scintigraphy. Bone scintigraphy is the most sensitive method for the assessment of bone metastasis, compared to clinical evaluation, bone radiographs, serum alkaline phosphatase, and prostatic acid phosphatase level [5]. Recent studies have shown that PET-CT is also highly sensitive and specific for the detection of bone metastasis [6].

Treatment Options

The therapeutic options for prostate cancer depend largely on the disease extent, while different functional and individual parameters (patient age, life expectancy, comorbidities) should also be taken into account [7]. Decision process should always be made in a multidisciplinary basis (including a urologist, radiation oncologist, and radiologist).

"Active Surveillance"

The concept of active surveillance was introduced in the past decade. It consists of an active decision not to treat the patient and follow him up with close surveillance and treat him only at predefined thresholds that define progression [7].

Validated "Curative" Treatment Options [7, 8]

- Radical prostatectomy: removal of the entire prostate gland and resection of both seminal vesicles along with sufficient surrounding tissue, so as to obtain a negative margin. Radical prostatectomy is performed with either conventional or robotic surgery.
- Radiation therapy: 3D conformal radiotherapy and intensity-modulated external beam radiotherapy is applied with good results in cases of localized and locally advanced PCa.
- Brachytherapy

All the above therapies are associated with relatively high morbidity rates, which mainly include incontinence, erectile dysfunction, and rectal toxicity [9, 10].

"Minimally Invasive" Ablation Therapies

A number of different minimally invasive ablation therapies have been introduced for the treatment of localized prostate cancer [7, 11–13]:
- Percutaneous Cryoablation
- High-Intensity Focused Ultrasound (HIFU)
- Photodynamic therapy
- Laser Ablation

Percutaneous Ablation Therapies for Prostate Cancer

Indications

1. Patients with organ-confined disease, or with minimal tumor extension beyond the prostate.
2. Prostate volume should be <40–50 mL
3. PSA-level <20 ngr/dL and biopsy Gleason score <7

Contraindications

Absolute

1. PSA-level >20 ngr/dL and biopsy Gleason score >7 (due to increased incidence of lymph node involvement)

Relative

1. Prior history of transurethral resection of the prostate (TURP), especially if there is a large transurethral defect present
2. Total gland volumes >50 mL (neoadjuvant cytoreduction with hormonal downsizing can be attempted in order to overcome the technical difficulty of treating large glands)
3. Uncorrectable coagulopathy

Laboratory Studies

The following should be obtained before the intervention:
1. Blood cells count (RBC, WBD, Platelets count)
2. Hemoglobin
3. INR

Percutaneous Prostate Cryoablation

Cryoablation tumor therapy consists of a series of steps in which tumors are repeatedly frozen and thawed [14–16]. Cryoablation causes tissue necrosis in situ based on three mechanisms:

- The extracellular and intracellular ice formation
- The osmolar effect of the ice crystals and finally
- The tissue ischemia

The basic principles of cryosurgery for tumors are fast cooling of the tissue to a lethal temperature, slow thawing, and repetition of the freeze – thaw cycle. Similar to other tissues, it has been proven, with in vitro experiments on cryoablation of prostatic adenocarcinoma cells that the lower the final temperature and the higher the freezing rate, the greater is the tissue necrosis achieved [17].

Image Guidance Modality

- Transrectal US-guidance:
  Transrectal US-probes are used for real-time transperineal placement of the cryoprobes into the prostate gland and monitoring of the freezing process [12, 18, 19].

Significant advances have been introduced regarding the transrectal US technology. Better imaging quality and use of duplex Doppler color is nowadays possible. Recently, the biplane ultrasound probes have been introduced. The above systems have two crystals that provide true cross-sectional and longitudinal imaging of the prostate [20].

The main limitation of the US-guidance is the poor monitoring of the ablation zone during the freezing process, due to the critical angle-shadowing effect of the ice-ball [20]. Only the proximal ice-ball edge is seen as a hyperechoic line, while the majority of the ablated area cannot be visualized.

- MR-guidance:

The transperineal probe positioning in the prostatic parenchyma can be done using real-time MR sequences (TRUFI SP, BEAT). During the freezing process, multiplanar real-time and high-resolution MR images are obtained for precise visualization of the ablation zone. The ice-ball is a signal void area on all conventional sequences, while the boundaries between the frozen and nonfrozen areas are depicted with excellent contrast. The use of real-time MR-temperature mapping allows the protection of the surrounding normal tissue (i.e. neurovascular bundle) from thermal injury.

Equipment

The equipment is similar as to any percutaneous cryoablation procedure:

- *Cryoprobes:* The third-generation cryoprobes are used today. The Seednet Cryomachine (Galil Medical, Yokneam, Israel) provides three different types of 17-G cryoprobes with a presumed ice-ball size and configuration. The cryoprobes can be placed directly without the use of an insertion coaxial system.
- *Urethral warming system:* The use of a urethral warming system is advised in order to protect the urethra mucosa [21]. These double-lumen catheters circulate warm saline solution colored with methylene blue. The catheters are directly connected to a circulating pump and a warmer. Warm saline (38–39.5°C) is circulated at a rate of 350 mL/min.
- *Rectal wall warming systems:* As for the urethra, a similar homemade warming system can be used for the rectum for rectal wall protection.
- *21-G spinal needle:* For dissection of the Denonvilliers fascia (in order to increase the distance between the prostate and the anterior rectal wall).
- *Thermosensors:* Different thermosensors can be used for real-time thermometry, in order to protect healthy structures from thermal injury (i.e. anterior rectal wall, neurovascular bundle).

Anesthesia

General or spinal anesthesia is required.

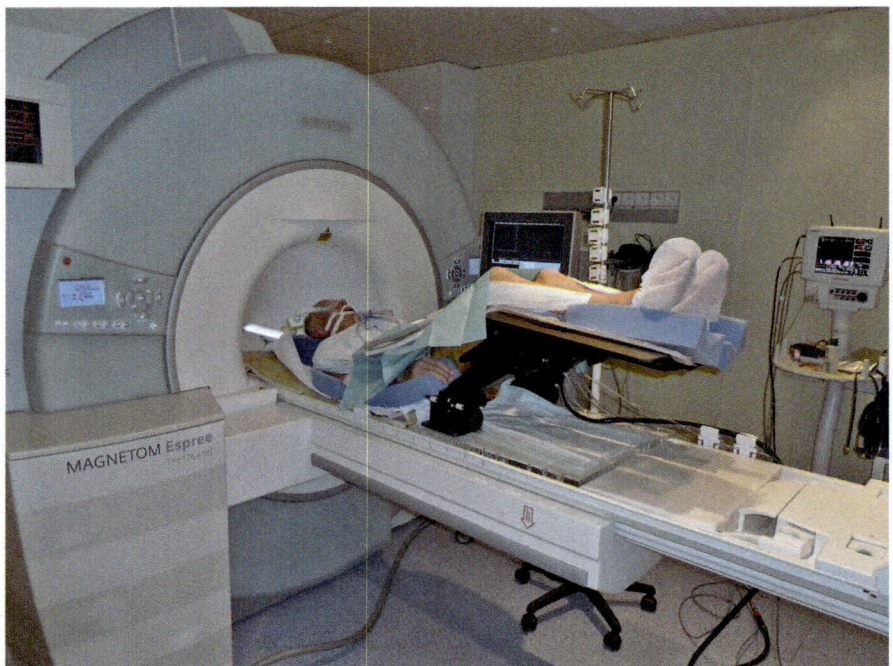

Fig. 13.1 Patient positioning for the percutaneous transperineal prostate cryoablation under MR-guidance. The patient is placed on the MR-table in supine position with the legs elevated using a homemade leg-support (in a gynecological position) exposing the perineum

Procedure Details

- The patient is placed on the table in a supine position with the legs elevated exposing the perineum, in a gynecological position (Fig. 13.1). A strip is used to elevate the scrotum out of the perineum. The perineum is then prepared and draped in a sterile manner.
- The cryoprobes are positioned through skin opening on the perineum. Probe positioning can be done using a free-hand technique, or with the use of a dedicated template (transrectal US-guidance). When MR-guidance is used, real-time T2W-Trufi images (in an axial and coronal to the cryoprobe plane) are used for the probe positioning. At the end of each needle positioning, a T2W-Blade sequence is obtained to reduce the needle artifact and to confirm the precise needle location within the gland. Probes are positioned with 1 cm distance and within 5 mm from the prostate capsule (Fig. 13.2).
- Once all cryoprobes are in place, the protective systems are positioned.
- Freezing process: Two 10-min freezing cycles separated by a 10-min passive thawing cycle are performed systematically. Ice-ball and temperature monitoring is mandatory during the freezing cycles (Fig. 13.3). The real-time temperature feedback on the anterior rectal wall should always be >16°C.

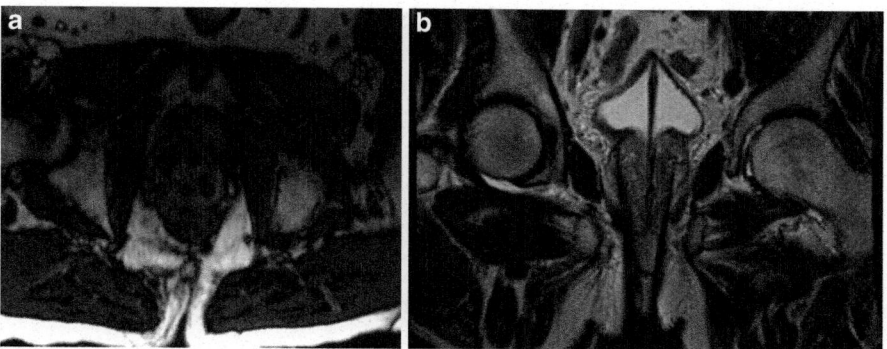

Fig. 13.2 Prostate cryoablation under MR-guidance. (**a**) Axial real-time T2W Trufi-image after positioning of six cryoprobes (Ice-rod) (before freezing), (**b**) Coronal high-resolution T2W Blade-image. Note the divergent orientation of the probes, according to the prostate pyramidal configuration

- Probes position can be readjusted (advanced or retrieved) whenever ice-ball configuration is considered inadequate to cover the total prostate gland volume.
- Whenever the ice-ball is approaching the rectal wall, or the real-time temperature feedback dropped below the safety margin (16°C), the corresponding cryoprobe can be manually slowed down or even stopped.

Endpoint

All probes should be stopped once the second 10-min freezing cycle is completed.

Immediate Postprocedure Care

- The perineum is controlled for case of hematoma.
- The urethra warming system is exchanged with a simple urethra catheter, which is kept in place for 24–48 h more.

Follow-Up

- The patients should be followed up at 3, 6, and 12 months after treatment, every 6 months thereafter until 3 years, and then annually, with clinical examination and PSA-level.

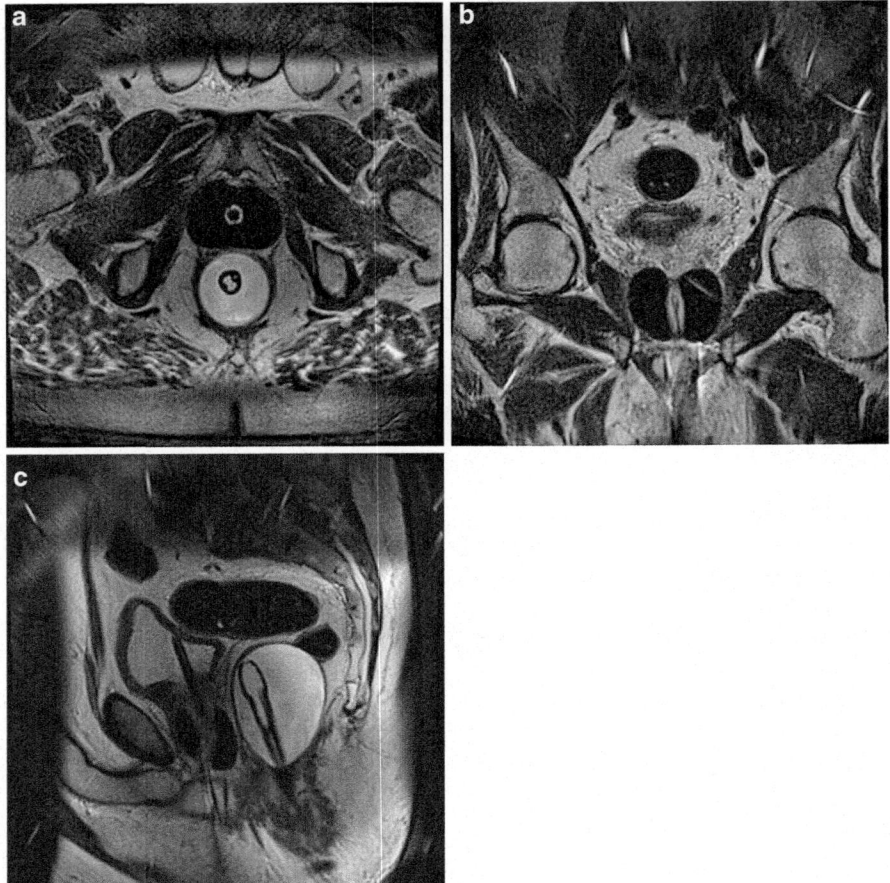

Fig. 13.3 Prostate cryoablation in a 65-year-old patient with prostatic carcinoma (Gleason score 3+3). Six cryoprobes (Ice-rod) were positioned: (**a**) axial, (**b**) coronal, and (**c**) sagittal images at the end of the freezing-cycle showing the sharp visualization of the ice-ball. Note the urethral warming catheter, and the rectal warming balloon-system with the MR-compatible fiber-optic thermosensor fixed on its anterior wall

- A postablation MRI can be performed to ensure complete coverage of the prostate gland.
- Postablation biopsy is not routinely necessary, unless there is a suspicion of local recurrence.
- Routine bone scans are not recommended in asymptomatic patients. If a patient has bone pain, a bone scan should be considered irrespective of PSA level.

Results

Long et al. performed a retrospective analysis of the multicenter, pooled, cryoablation results of 975 patients stratified into three risk groups [22]. Using PSA thresholds of 1.0 ngr/mL and <0.5 ngr/mL at a mean follow-up of 24 months, the 5-year bio-chemical disease-free rate was:

- 76% and 60%, respectively, for the low-risk group
- 71% and 45%, respectively, for the intermediate-risk group
- 61% and 36%, respectively, for the high-risk group

With regard to third-generation cryoablation technology, clinical follow-up is short, with a 12-month follow-up available in 110/176 patients [22–27]. Of these, 80 patients (73%) have a PSA-nadir <0.4 ngr/mL.

In our department, percutaneous prostate cryoablation under MR-guidance was performed in 11 patients. The procedure was technically feasible in 10 out of 11 patients. Mean follow-up is 15 months (range: 1–25 months). Mean PSA-nadir is 0.33 ngr/mL (range: 0.02–0.94 ngr/mL).

Complications

- Erectile dysfunction (~80%)
- Tissue sloughing (3%)
- Incontinence (4.4%)
- Pelvic pain (1.4%)
- Urinary retention (2%)
- Fistula (<0.5%) [22–27]

HIFU of the Prostate

High-intensity focused ultrasound consists of focused ultrasound waves emitted from a transducer. The concentration of the beam energy at a specific point produces a dramatic temperature rise (up to 80°C in a few seconds) causing coagulation necrosis of the tissues. The volume of tissue destruction is small (1–3 mm in width, 5–20 mm in height); consequently, in order to destroy the entire tumor, it is necessary that elementary focal lesions be placed side-to-side throughout the targeted tissue [28, 29].

Regarding HIFU for prostate cancer: Transrectal US-guidance is used. The procedure is performed under general or spinal anesthesia. The patient is lying in a lateral position.

The procedure is time-consuming, with about 10 gr of prostatic tissue treated per hour [7].

Complications [7]

- Urinary retention is one of the most common complications developing in almost all patients

- Urinary incontinence (12%)
- Impotence (55–70%)
- Chronic pain
- Rectal anal fistulas

Results

The most successful HIFU treatments have been those that have ablated the whole gland. Success rates for the treatment of prostate cancer range from 60% [30] to 80% [31] of patients being disease-free at repeat biopsy and showing a reduction of serum PSA values <4 ngr/mL.

Photodynamic Therapy of the Prostate

Photodynamic therapy involves the activation of a photosensitizer by a specific wavelength of light in the presence of oxygen to create cell damage and tissue necrosis.

The photosensitizer is administered (orally or intravenously) in a stable inactive form. When it is exposed to light of a certain wavelength, the photosensitizer reaches a higher unstable energy state. In this unstable form, the activated photosensitizer releases energy by emitting heat, light, or converting to an intermediate energy state, prior to returning to a stable ground state.

The photosensitizing drugs are either activated while in the tissue, or in the vasculature. Tissue-activated drugs have long drug light intervals (hours to days). In contrast, the vascular-activated drugs have short drug light interval (min) and the whole treatment is done in a single session [13].

Light delivery to the prostate tissue is done by means of low-power laser light optical fibers. The fibers are positioned to the prostate using the transperineal approach.

Results

Results in the literature regarding the efficacy of photodynamic therapy are limited. Several authors report that around 60% of men receiving whole-gland treatment at a maximal drug and light dose have a complete response to treatment and negative prostate biopsy at 6 months follow-up [32–35].

Complications

- Erectile dysfunction
- Urinary incontinence
- Urethral strictures
- Bowel dysfunction

Laser Ablation of the Prostate

Laser interstitial thermal therapy uses laser light to deposit high-energy photons locally in tissue causing tissue destruction through rapid heating [36, 37]. Laser ablation has been used for the treatment of confined or recurred prostate cancer in nonsurgical candidates. In order to achieve larger ablation zones, the internally cooled diffusing-tip fiber-optic applicators should be preferred. The laser fibers are placed transperineally, using transrectal US- or MR-guidance (with the use of MR-compatible applicators).

Focal Therapy of the Prostate

During the last two decades, there has been a trend toward earlier diagnosis of the prostate cancer (greater public and professional awareness, screening test). Nowadays, more men with earlier cancer stages are identified.

The different ablative therapies described have been adopted to treat locally small, restricted tumors. With the focal therapy of the PCa, we intend to preserve the genitourinary function with adequate treatment of the tumor.

Indications [7]

1. Patients with low to moderate risk, tumor clinical stage ≤cT2a, and radiological stage ≤cT2a.

The patients should undergo a transperineal template mapping biopsy, to define exact tumor location, extent, prior treatment.

Contraindications [7]

1. Patients who have undergone radiation therapy of the prostate are not candidates.
2. Patients with previous prostate surgery should be counseled with caution.

When the option of focal therapy is considered, the patient should always be informed that the therapy is under evaluation and that there is a possibility of repeat (re-do) treatment [7].

References

1. Ferlay J, Autier P, Boniol M, Heanue M, Colombet M, Boyle P. Estimates of the cancer incidence and mortality in Europe in 2006. Ann Oncol. 2007;18:581–92.
2. Jemal A, Siegel R, Xu J, Ward E. Cancer statistics. CA Cancer J Clin. 2010;60:277–300.
3. Parkin DM, Bray FI, Devesa SS. Cancer burden in the year 2000: the global picture. Eur J Cancer. 2001;37 Suppl 8:S4–66.
4. Claus FG, Hricak H, Hattery RR. Pretreatment evaluation of prostate cancer: role of MR imaging and 1H MR Spectroscopy. Radiographics. 2004;24:S167.
5. McGregor B, Tulloch AG, Quinlan MF, Lovegrove F. The role of bone scanning in the assessment of prostatic carcinoma. Br J Urol. 1978;50:178–81.
6. Beheshti M, Vali R, Langsteger W. 18 F-Fluorocholine PET-CT in the assessment of bone metastases in prostate cancer. Eur J Nucl Med Mol Imaging. 2007;34:1316–7.
7. Heidenreich A, Bellmunt J, Bolla M, et al. European Association of Urology guidelines on prostate cancer. Part 1: screening, diagnosis, and treatment of clinically localised disease. Eur Urol. 2011;59:61–71.
8. Salembier C, Lavagnini P, Nickers P, GEC ESTRO PROBATE Group, et al. Tumour target volumes in permanent prostate brachytherapy: a supplement to the ESTRO/EAU/EORTC recommendations on prostate brachytherapy. Radiother Oncol. 2007;83:3–10.
9. Potosky AL, Legler J, Albertsen PC, et al. Health outcomes after prostatectomy or radiotherapy for prostate cancer: results from the Prostate Cancer Outcome Study. J Natl Cancer Inst. 2000;92:1582–92.
10. Ataman F, Zurlo A, Artignan X, et al. Late toxicity following conventional radiotherapy for prostate cancer: analysis of the EORTC trial 22863. Eur J Cancer. 2004;40:1674–81.
11. Onik G, Narayan P, Vaughan D, Dineen M, Brunelle R. Focal "nerve-sparing" cryosurgery for treatment of primary prostate cancer: a new approach to preserving potency. Urology. 2002;60:109–14.
12. Onik G. Percutaneous image-guided prostate cancer treatment: cryoablation as a successful example. Tech Vasc Interv Radiol. 2007;10:149–58.
13. Ahmed HU, Moore C, Emberton M. Minimally-invasive technologies in uro-oncology: the role of cryotherapy, HIFU and photodynamic therapy in whole gland and focal therapy of localised prostate cancer. Surg Oncol. 2009;18:219–32.
14. Theodorescu D. Cancer cryotherapy: evolution and biology. Rev Urol. 2004;6 Suppl 4:S9–19.
15. Mazur P. Cryobiology: the freezing of biological systems. Science. 1970;68:939–49.
16. Mazur P. The role of intracellular freezing in the death of cells cooled at supraoptimal rates. Cryobiology. 1977;14:251–72.

17. Tatsutani K, Rubinsky B, Onik G, Dahiya R. Effect of thermal variables on frozen human primary prostatic adenocarcinoma cells. Urology. 1996;48:441–7.
18. Onik G. Image-guided prostate cryosurgery: state of the art. Cancer Control. 2001;8:522–31.
19. Onik GM, Cohen JK, Reyes GD, Rubinsky B, Chang Z, Baust J. Transrectal ultrasound-guided percutaneous radical cryosurgical ablation of the prostate. Cancer. 1993;72:1291–9.
20. Saliken JC, Donnelly BJ, Rewcastle JC. The evolution and state of modern technology for prostate cryosurgery. Urology. 2002;60(Suppl 2A):26–33.
21. Cohen JK, Miller RJ, Shuman BA. Urethral warming catheter for use during cryoablation of the prostate. Urology. 1995;45:861–4.
22. Long JP, Bahn D, Lee F, Shinohara K, Chinn DO, Macaluso Jr JN. Five-year retrospective, multi-institutional pooled analysis of cancer-related outcomes after cryosurgical ablation of the prostate. Urology. 2001;57:518–23.
23. Han KR, Cohen JK, Miller RJ, et al. Treatment of organ confined prostate cancer with third generation cryosurgery: preliminary multicenter experience. J Urol. 2003;170:1126–30.
24. Koppie TM, Shinohara K, Grossfeld GD, Presti Jr JC, Carroll PR. The efficacy of cryosurgical ablation of prostate cancer: the University of California, San Francisco experience. J Urol. 1999;162:427–32.
25. De La Taille A, Benson MC, Bagiella E, et al. Cryoablation for clinically localized prostate cancer using an argon-based system: complication rates and biochemical recurrence. BJU Int. 2000;85:281–6.
26. Donelly BJ, Saliken JC, Ernst DS, et al. Prospective trial of cryosurgical ablation of the prostate: five-year results. Urology. 2002;60:645–9.
27. Bahn DK, Lee F, Badalament R, Kumar A, Greski J, Chernick M. Targeted cryoablation of the prostate: 7-year outcomes in the primary treatment of prostate cancer. Urology. 2002;60:3–11.
28. Rouviere O, Souchon R, Salomir R, Gelet A, Chapelon J-Y, Luonnet D. Tranrectal high-intensity focused ultrasound ablation of prostate cancer: effective treatment requiring accurate imaging. Eur J Radiol. 2007;63:317–27.
29. Zhoux YF. High-intensity focused ultrasound in clinical tumor ablation. World J Clin Oncol. 2011;2:8–27.
30. Gelet A, Chapelon JY, Bouvier R, et al. Transrectal high-intensity focused ultrasound: minimally invasive therapy of localised prostate cancer. J Endourol. 2000;14:519–28.
31. Chaussy C, Thuroff S. High-intensity focused ultrasound in prostate cancer: results after 3 years. Mol Urol. 2000;4:179–82.
32. Weersink RA, Forbes J, Bisland S, et al. Assessment of cutaneous photosensitivity of TOOKAD (WST09) in preclinical animal models and patients. Photochem Photobiol. 2005;81:106–13.
33. Trachtenberg J, Weersink RA, Davidson SR, et al. Vascular-targeted photodynamic therapy (padoporfin, WST09) for recurrent prostate cancer after failure of external beam radiotherapy: a study of escalating light doses. BJU Int. 2008;102:556–62.
34. Trachtenberg J, Bogaards A, Weersink RA, et al. Vascular targeted photodynamic therapy with palladium-bacteriopheophorbide photosensitizer for recurrent prostate cancer following definitive radiation therapy; assessment of safety and treatment response. J Urol. 2007;178:1974–9.
35. Haider MA, Davidson SR, Kale AV, et al. Prostate gland: MR imaging apperance after vascular targeted photodynamic therapy with palladium-bacteriopheophorbide. Radiology. 2007;244:196–204.
36. Woodrum DA, Mynderse LA, Gorny KR, Amrami KK, McNichols RJ, Callstrom MR. 3.0 T MR-guided laser ablation of a prostate cancer recurrence in the postsurgical prostate bed. J Vasc Interv Radiol. 2011;22:929–34.
37. Linder U, Lawrentschuk N, Trachtenberg J. Focal laser ablation for localized prostate cancer. J Endourol. 2010;24:791–7.

Chapter 14
Ablation of Primary Bone and Soft Tissue Tumors

Konstantinos Katsanos and Theodore Petsas

Osteoid Osteoma

Background Facts

- Osteoid osteoma (OO) is a benign skeletal neoplasm of unknown etiology consisting of both osteoid and woven bone elements that are surrounded by osteoblasts. Vascularized lesion was clearly separate from reactive woven or lamellar bone.
- OO represents 4% of all bone tumors and accounts for 12% of all benign cases. The lesion is usually smaller than 1.5 cm in diameter and may occur in any bone, but afflicts the appendicular skeleton in approximately two thirds of the patients. Neuroaxial location in approximately 6% of the cases.
- Dull or aching pain, worse during the night, typically relieved by salicylates (Aspirin) and nonsteroidal anti-inflammatory drugs (NSAIDs). Pain attributed to local release of prostaglandins (PGE2 and 6-keto-PGF1α) leading to a chronic inflammatory response and subsequent periosteal reaction and synovitis.
- Usual appearance is of a small sclerotic bone island within a circular lucent defect called a nidus. The central radiolucent nidus is surrounded by considerable cortical and endosteal bone sclerosis.

K. Katsanos, M.Sc., M.D., Ph.D., EBIR (✉)
T. Petsas, M.D., Ph.D.
Department of Interventional Radiology,
Patras University Hospital (PGNP),
Panepistimiou Street, Rion, Patras 26504, Greece
e-mail: katsanos@med.upatras.gr;
petsas@med.upatras.gr

T. Clark, T. Sabharwal (eds.), *Interventional Radiology Techniques in Ablation*,
Techniques in Interventional Radiology,
DOI 10.1007/978-0-85729-094-6_14, © Springer-Verlag London 2013

Fig. 14.1 Image from the past. Typical CT features of an osteoid osteoma located in the posterior upper tibia (*vertical white arrow*). Note the characteristic nidus surrounded by dense sclerotic bone. *Wide horizontal white arrow* denotes an unsuccessful previous attempt of surgical curettage

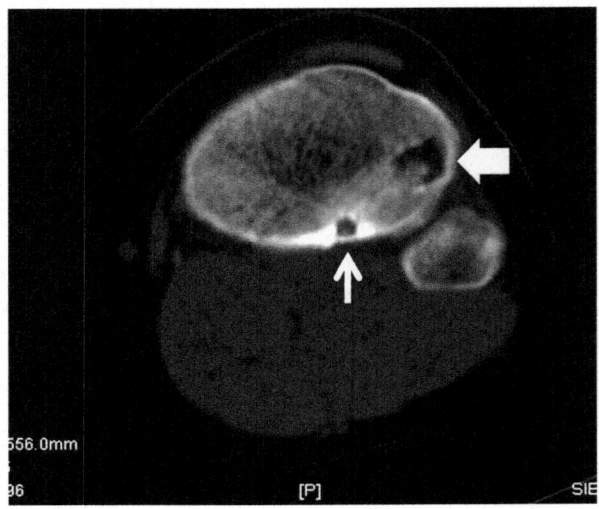

Alternative Therapies

- Tumor ablation is indicated in cases of failure, contraindication, or intolerance to conventional medical pain management. Prolonged presence of the painful tumor may lead to osteoarthritis, spinal deformity, or disturbed growth of the extremities.
- Orthopedic surgical en bloc resection or bone curettage with/without bone graft replacement (Fig. 14.1). Arthroscopic removal for intra-articular lesions has been reported. Surgical resection has an 88–95% success rate, 20–30% minor complication rate, and 3.0–4.5% incidence of major complications (e.g. fractures).
- Spontaneous regression within 2–8 years without treatment has been reported, probably because of infarction of the tumor feeding vessel.

Imaging Features

- There is typically an intracortical nidus with fusiform cortical thickening, reactive sclerosis, and variable surrounding bone marrow edema.
- Depending on lesion size and anatomy, a combination of plain radiography, computed tomography (CT), gadolinium-enhanced MRI, or radionuclide bone scan may be necessary to adequately characterize tumor morphology.
- Plain radiography is the initial examination of choice and usually shows a radiolucent nidus surrounded by extensive cortical bone thickening.
- Typical MRI features include extensive bone marrow edema with focal contrast uptake.
- Nuclear imaging scans usually show focal intense uptake of the radionuclide corresponding to the site of tumor location.

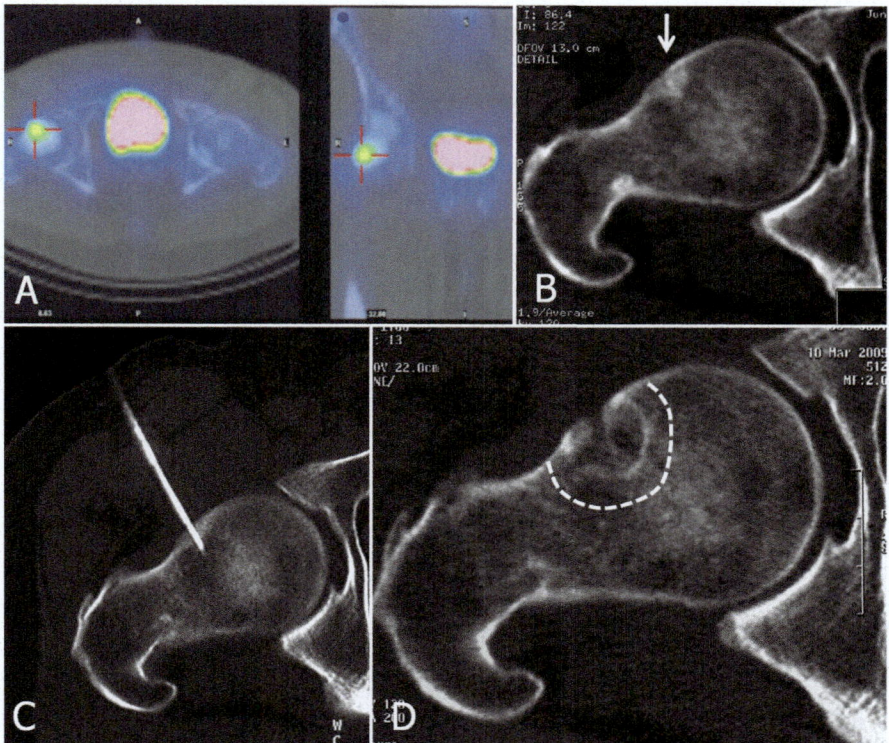

Fig. 14.2 Percutaneous RF ablation of OO. (**a**) SPECT scintigraphic imaging shows intense radiotracer uptake in case of an OO located in the right femoral head. (**b**) In conjunction with the scintigraphic information, thin-section CT pinpoints the exact location of the lesion with atypical features (*white arrow*). (**c**) CT-guided introduction of an RF electrode permits accurate placement of the needle inside the target-nidus. (**d**) Follow-up after 1 year shows a well-defined area of bone necrosis surrounded by reactive sclerosis (*dotted white line*). The patient remains free of symptoms

- Thin-section CT with multiplanar reformatting (VRT, MIP, and MPR reconstructions) and/or single-photon emission tomography (SPECT) may help in precisely pinpointing the location of the tumor (Fig. 14.2).

Differential Diagnosis

- Bone island, old infarct, stress fracture callus, chronic or healed osteomyelitis.
- Osteoblastoma, chondroblastoma, ossifying fibroma, enchondroma.
- Digital subtraction angiography may differentiate the tumor from a Brodie abscess.
- Painful intracortical chondroma has been described as a rare differential diagnosis. It may also be treated with radiofrequency ablation.

Patient Preparation and Anesthesia

- Obtain informed consent as necessary
- Obtain baseline labs – evaluate for infection or sepsis
- Evaluate platelet count and coagulation parameters.
- Discontinue clopidogrel, aspirin, and NSAIDs as necessary/5–10 days in case of neuroaxial procedures
- Adhere to strict sterility practice, as in all muskuloskeletal procedures
- Antibiotic prophylaxis with a second- or third-generation cephalosporin. May be continued per os after the procedure.

Contraindications

- Uncooperative patient
- Uncorrectable coagulopathy
- Inability to safely access the lesion
- Systemic infection or sepsis

Image Guidance and Lesion Access

- Computed tomography (CT) is the imaging method of choice for precise localization of the OO nidus and accurate guidance during percutaneous thermal ablation. CT has high spatial resolution that is critical for the targeting of difficult-to-access neuroaxial lesions.
- After careful review of the thin-section CT scan, the needle path transversing the least thickness of corticol bone must be chosen. In case of long bones, access from the contralateral side may help stabilize the trocar/needle within the diaphysis.
- Angling of the computed tomography scanner gantry may aid accessibility if traditional orthogonal axial views fail to show a safe route of access.
- CT fluoroscopy is an emerging adjunctive tool for high-precision real-time guided targeting of subtle lesions. Scanning parameters must be carefully adjusted to minimize radiation exposure.

Ablation Technique

- Thermoablation of OOs was first reported in the early 1990s.

- Intervention is performed under general or spinal anesthesia, because penetration and ablation of the OO nidus is extremely painful. Nerve blocks can be used if the extremities are involved.
- Lesion access with a durable bone trocar of appropriate diameter; e.g. 10–15G vertebroplasty trocars with diamond- or bevel-shaped needles. Use a sterile hammer to introduce the bone trocar and orientate the bevel of the trocar as necessary to adjust the needle pathway. Image-guided drilling may be required to gain access through dense cortical bone.
- Once access has been gained, standard bone biopsy is obtained with use of appropriate trephine trocars. If possible, sampling of more than one specimen is encouraged.
- Thermoablation with interstitial laser photocoagulation (laser optical fiber) or standard radiofrequency device (nonperfused radiofrequency electrode). Co-axial insertion of the electrode device through the bone cannula.
- After successful placement of the electrode, withdraw the cannula as much as possible without displacing the electrode. Direct contact of the metal cannula with the active electrode tip may overheat the cannula and result in soft tissue and skin burns.
- Radiofrequency ablation parameters: Commercial RF generator, nonperfused monopolar electrode, length of active electrode tip 7–10 mm, effective power <10 W (usually 3–5 W), target temperature 90–95°C, duration of 5–10 min, limited by vaporization and/or carbonization in case of >100°C.
- In case of laser photocoagulation, thermoablation is produced with near-infrared wavelengths lasers (neodymium yttrium aluminum garnet Nd:YAG).

Thermal Monitoring and Organ Insulation

- Monitoring of local temperature increase is crucial in case of neuroaxial OOs with sensitive adjacent anatomical structures, such as the spinal cord and exiting nerve roots.
- One or more thermocouples may be employed for continuous thermal monitoring of the anatomy of interest. Single thermocouples are available as 21G needles inserted under routine image guidance in proximity with the lesion of interest.
- Thermal insulating techniques like carbon dioxide insufflations may decrease heat conductivity between the source electrode and other sensitive organs of interest. Epidural carbon dioxide infusions have been described.
- Whenever applying thermal ablative therapies in the skeleton, beware of the electrode being close to metal implants or other metallic osteosynthetic materials, because of their high electrical and heat energy conductance.

Treatment Outcomes

- Immediate postprocedural pain may be significant; NSAIDs and narcotics as necessary.
- Majority of patients report resolution of pain symptoms after 24–48 h.
- <10% of the patients become symptom-free after 1–2 weeks.
- Reactive sclerosis of the ablated lesions is evident on CT/MR after a period of 6 months to 2 years.
- Overall clinical success rates vary from around 80% to almost 100%.
- Late local recurrence is 5–6%; best treated with repeat thermoablation.

Complications

- Local hematoma. Bleeding or hemorrhage is usually self-limited.
- Synovitis, arthritis, fluid collection in case of intra-articular OOs
- Neurodystrophia, Sudeck's atrophy

Other Bone and Soft Tissue Tumors

Osteoblastomas

Background Facts

- Osteoblastomas account for only 0.5–2% of all primary bone tumors and only 3% of benign bone tumors. Almost 90% of the cases are diagnosed before the age of 30 years.
- Osteoblastomas share the same clinical and histologic manifestations with OOs; therefore, some consider the two tumors to be variants of the same disease, with osteoblastoma representing a giant osteoid osteoma.
- Expansile lesions with a sclerotic or shell-like rim. Located in the spine in 30–40% of the cases, usually afflict the posterior spinal elements.
- Osteoblastomas may exhibit aggressive behavior and exceed a diameter of 2 cm. They may recur after initially successful thermoablation.
- The same principles of OO ablation account also for radiofrequency ablation of osteoblastomas (Fig. 14.3).
- Depending on lesion size, electrodes with a longer active tip, needle repositioning, and multiple ablation sessions may be required. Do not forget bone biopsy for histological confirmation.

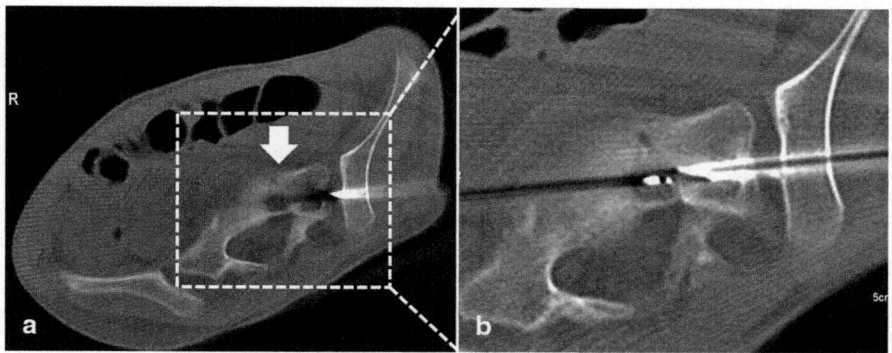

Fig. 14.3 Osteoblastoma thermoablation. (**a**) CT-guided insertion of a 10-G beveled bone trocar to target an osteoblastoma of the sacrum in a 13-year-old female patient suffering from excruciating pain. The trocar was inserted through the iliac bone and the sacroiliac joint (fibrous part) to avoid any damage of the sensitive neurovascular structures. (**b**) Note the co-axial insertion of a nonperfused RF electrode with a 1-cm long active tip inside the nidus of the lesion. Three ablative sessions, each 5–10 min long, were delivered with the electrode in slightly different orientations to cover the whole lesion. Epidural placement of a thermocouple to monitor the temperature around the adjacent descending sacral roots would be recommended. Pain resolved completely after 1 week and the girl remains free of symptoms for 2 years now

Chondroblastomas

- Chondroblastoma is a rare cartilaginous bone tumor; accounts for 1% of bone tumors. It originates from chondroblasts, hence the name.
- It is the most common epiphyseal tumor during childhood. It is usually benign with a slow-growing nature.
- Usually afflicts the epiphysis of immature long bones prohibiting surgical resection. The knee area and proximal humerus are involved in around 70% of the cases.
- The same principles of OO ablation account also for radiofrequency ablation of chondroblastomas. Depending on lesion size, needle repositioning and multiple ablation sessions may be required. Do not forget bone biopsy for histological confirmation. Chondroblastoma must be differentiated from clear-cell chondrosarcoma.
- Only small successful series still reported in the literature. Radiofrequency produced heat may damage the nearby joint cartilage and lead to arthritis compromising the joint function.

Other Applications

- Radiofrequency ablation has been also successfully applied for the eradication of giant cell tumors, enchondromas, eosinophilic granulomas, bone hemangiomas, and intracortical chondromas. However, relevant reports in the literature remain scarce.

- There are isolated reports of radiofrequency ablation of inoperable or unresectable recurrent tumors like sacral chordomas and soft tissue sarcomas. However, thermoablation in such extraordinary cases must be part of a multidisciplinary treatment protocol encompassing surgery, chemotherapy, and radiation therapy.
- Desmoid tumors are infiltrative fibroblastic benign neoplasms that tend to recur locally after surgical excision and show poor response to irradiation and chemotherapy. Percutaneous chemical or thermal ablative techniques may be efficacious in the eradication and/or local control of these aggressive tumors.
- Although radiofrequency is the leading multipurpose tool for ablation of the skeletal system, other technologies such as cryoablation or high-intensity focused ultrasound (HIFU) may be considered.

Key Points

- OO is a benign skeletal neoplasm of unknown etiology consisting of both osteoid and woven bone. It represents 4% of all bone tumors and accounts for 12% of all benign cases. The lesion is usually smaller than 1.5 cm in diameter and produces dull or aching pain, worse during the night, typically relieved by salicylates (Aspirin).
- Depending on lesion size and anatomy, a combination of plain radiography, CT, gadolinium-enhanced MRI, or radionuclide bone scan may be necessary to adequately characterize tumor morphology. OOs are typically characterized by an intracortical nidus with fusiform cortical thickening, reactive sclerosis, and variable surrounding bone marrow edema.
- OOs are one of the best indications for minimally invasive percutaneous thermoablation. Radiofrequency ablation for OOs is performed under general anesthesia and computed tomography guidance with excellent clinical results and minimal complications.
- Radiofrequency ablation has been also successfully applied for the eradication of osteoblastomas, chondroblastomas, giant cell tumors, enchondromas, eosinophilic granulomas, bone hemangiomas, and intracortical chondromas. Cytoreduction of sacral chordomas and sarcomas, and local control of aggressive desmoid tumors with percutaneous ablative methods have been also reported.

Suggested Reading

Gangi A, Tsoumakidou G, Buy X, Quoix E. Quality improvement guidelines for bone tumour management. Cardiovasc Intervent Radiol. 2010;33(4):706–13.

Kujak JL, Liu PT, Johnson GB, Callstrom MR. Early experience with percutaneous cryoablation of extra-abdominal desmoid tumors. Skeletal Radiol. 2010;39(2):175–82.

Petsas T, Megas P, Papathanassiou Z. Radiofrequency ablation of two femoral head chondroblastomas. Eur J Radiol. 2007;63(1):63–7. Epub 2007 May 4.

Sabharwal T, Katsanos K, Buy X, Gangi A. Image-guided ablation therapy of bone tumors. Semin Ultrasound CT MR. 2009;30(2):78–90.

Welch BT, Welch TJ. Percutaneous ablation of benign bone tumors. Tech Vasc Interv Radiol. 2011;14(3):118–23.

Index

The manufacturer's authorised representative in the EU is Springer
Nature Customer Service Centre GmbH, Europaplatz 3, 69115 Heidelberg,
Germany. If you have any concerns regarding our products, please
contact ProductSafety@springernature.com

Printed and bound by CPI Group (UK) Ltd, Croydon, CR0 4YY

23/04/2026

02095604-0003